KU-375-516

An Atlas of Investigation and Management

INFLAMMATORY BOWEL DISEASE

An Atlas of Investigation and Management

INFLAMMATORY BOWEL DISEASE

Timothy R Orchard
Consultant Physician and Gastroenterologist, and Reader in Gastroenterology
Gastroenterology Unit, St. Mary's Hospital
Imperial College Healthcare NHS Trust
London, UK

Robert D Goldin
Consultant Histopathologist
Department of Histopathology, St. Mary's Hospital
Imperial College Healthcare NHS Trust
London, UK

Paris P Tekkis
Consultant Surgeon and Reader in Surgery
Chelsea and Westminster Hospital
London, UK

Horace RT Williams
Consultant Physician and Gastroenterologist
Gastroenterology Unit, St. Mary's Hospital
Imperial College Healthcare NHS Trust
London, UK

CLINICAL PUBLISHING

OXFORD

Clinical Publishing
an imprint of Atlas Medical Publishing Ltd
Oxford Centre for Innovation
Mill Street, Oxford OX2 0JX, UK

Tel: +44 1865 811116
Fax: +44 1865 251550
Email: info@clinicalpublishing.co.uk
Web: www.clinicalpublishing.co.uk

Distributed in USA and Canada by:
Clinical Publishing
30 Amberwood Parkway
Ashland, OH 44805, USA

Tel: 800-247-6553 (toll free within US and Canada)
Fax: 419-281-6883
Email: order@bookmasters.com

Distributed in UK and Rest of World by:
Marston Book Services Ltd
PO Box 269
Abingdon
Oxon OX14 4YN, UK

Tel: +44 1235 465500
Fax: +44 1235 465555
Email: trade.orders@marston.co.uk

MONXLANDS HOSPITAL
LIBRARY
MONKSCOURT AVENUE
AIRDRIE ML60IS
☎ 01236712005

© Atlas Medical Publishing Ltd 2011

First published 2011

All rights reserved. No part of this publication may be reproduced, stored in a retrieval system, or transmitted, in any form or by any means, without the prior permission in writing of Clinical Publishing or Atlas Medical Publishing Ltd.

Although every effort has been made to ensure that all owners of copyright material have been acknowledged in this publication, we would be glad to acknowledge in subsequent reprints or editions any omissions brought to our attention.

A catalogue record of this book is available from the British Library

ISBN print   978 1 84692 013 4
ISBN e-book 978 1 84692 506 1

The publisher makes no representation, express or implied, that the dosages in this book are correct. Readers must therefore always check the product information and clinical procedures with the most up-to-date published product information and data sheets provided by the manufacturers and the most recent codes of conduct and safety regulations. The authors and the publisher do not accept any liability for any errors in the text or for the misuse or misapplication of material in this work.

Printed by Henry Ling, Dorchester Press, Dorset, UK

Contents

Contributors

David Walker
Clinical Research Fellow
Imperial College London
London, UK

Nicholas Powell
Hon. Specialist Registrar
Imperial College Healthcare NHS Trust
London, UK

Evangelos Russo
Clinical Research Fellow
Imperial College London
London, UK

Julie Cornish
Clinical Research Fellow
Department of Surgery
Imperial College London
London, UK

Abbreviations

5-ASA 5-aminosalicylic acid
6-MP 6-mercaptopurine
ALM adenoma-like dysplastic lesion or mass
AS ankylosing spondylitis
ASGE American Society of Gastrointestinal Endoscopy
AXR abdominal X-ray
Aza azathioprine
BSG British Society of Gastroenterology
CARD caspase recruitment domain
CD Crohn's disease
CDT *Clostridium difficile* toxin
CMV cytomegalovirus
CRC colorectal cancer

CREST (syndrome) Calcinosis, Raynaud's syndrome, oEsophageal dysmotility, Sclerodactyly and Telangiectasia (syndrome)
CRP C-reactive protein
CT computed tomography
DALM dysplasia-associated lesion/mass
DNA deoxyribonucleic acid
EIM extraintestinal manifestation
EN erythema nodosum
ERCP endoscopic retrograde cholangiopancreatography
ESR erythrocyte sedimentation rate
EUS endoscopic ultrasound
FDR first degree relative
Foxp3 forkhead box protein 3

GI gastrointestinal

HLA human leukocyte antigen

HSG hysterosalpingography

IBD inflammatory bowel disease

IBDU inflammatory bowel disease, type unclassified

IFN-γ interferon-γ

Il interleukin

IPAA ileal pouch anal anastamosis (a form of RPC)

IRGM immunity-related guanosine triphosphatase family, M

iv intravenous

IVF *in vitro* fertilization

LBW low birth weight

MAP *Mycobacterium avium paratuberculosis*

MCP metacarpophalangeal

MC&S microscopy, culture, and sensitivity

MMR measles mumps and rubella vaccine

MMX multimatrix

MRCP magnetic resonance cholangiopancreatography

MRI magnetic resonance imaging

NBI narrow band imaging

NF-κB, Nuclear factor kappa-light-chain-enhancer of activated B cells

NICE National Institute for Health and Clinical Excellence

NOD nucleotide-binding oligomerization domain

NSAID nonsteroidal anti-inflammatory drug

OCTN organic cation transporter

OGD oesophago-gastro-duodenoscopy

PG pyoderma gangrenosum

PSC primary sclerosing cholangitis

RNA ribonucleic acid

PPARγ peroxisome proliferator-activated receptor gamma

qds (quater die sumendus) Latin: four times a day

RPC restorative proctocolectomy (usually synonymous with IPAA)

STAT-3 signal transducer and activator of transcription 3

STC subtotal colectomy

TB tuberculosis

TGF-β transforming growth factor-β

Th (cell) T helper (cell)

TNF tumour necrosis factor

TPMT thiopurine methyltransferase

Treg regulatory T cell

UC ulcerative colitis

UDCA ursodeoxycholic acid

UP ulcerative proctitis

US ultrasonography

VTE venous thromboembolism

WBC white blood cell count

Part 1

DIAGNOSIS AND MANAGEMENT OF INFLAMMATORY BOWEL DISEASE

Chapter 1

Introduction: aetiology and clinical presentation

DIFFERENCES BETWEEN CROHN'S DISEASE AND ULCERATIVE COLITIS

The term inflammatory bowel disease (IBD) is generally used to describe ulcerative colitis (UC) and Crohn's disease (CD), chronic idiopathic disorders characterized by gastrointestinal (GI) inflammation. CD can affect any part of the alimentary tract while UC affects only the large bowel. The prevalence of IBD is approximately 230 per 100,000 population in the western world, with an incidence of 15 per 100,000 per year. In 5–10% of cases there is clinical and endoscopic evidence for chronic colonic IBD but no definitive histological evidence to favour either CD or UC, and such patients are said to have indeterminate colitis, a term recently updated to inflammatory bowel disease, type unclassified (IBDU). In both conditions inflammation may occur at sites distant to the gut, so called extraintestinal manifestions. These may include arthritis, primary sclerosing cholangitis, ocular and cutaneous inflammation. The pathogenesis of IBD has not yet been fully elucidated, but it is thought to involve an abnormal, genetically predetermined response to an environmental trigger which is likely to be bacterial.

CD and UC may have similar symptoms, but distinguishing between the conditions is important due to differences in prognosis and management. Medical therapies are instigated to induce and maintain remission, and the efficacy of these may differ between the two conditions. Unfortunately surgical options may become necessary and the course of disease differs between UC and CD: 15–40% of those with UC will eventually come to colectomy, while between two-thirds and three-quarters of those with CD will require surgery at some time, and of these 50% will require a second operation. A colectomy for UC is generally considered to be curative; this is not the case for CD.

The main differences between CD and UC are summarized in *Table 1.1*. It should be noted that these are generalizations, and that more detailed explanations can be found elsewhere in the book.

Table 1.1 Main differences between CD and UC

Crohn's disease		*Ulcerative colitis*	
Location		*Location*	
Any part of the alimentary tract affected:		Only large bowel affected (though possibility of 'backwash ileitis'):	
	Cases (%)		Cases (%)
Ileocolonic	45	Proctitis	25
Colitis only	25	Left-sided (to splenic flexure)	45
Terminal ileum only	20	Extensive / pancolitis	30
Extensive small bowel	5		
Anorectal only	3		
Other (gastroduodenal, oral)	2		
Clinical		*Clinical*	
Diarrhoea +/- rectal bleeding		Diarrhoea	
Weight loss		Rectal bleeding	
Abdominal pain			
Constitutional symptoms			
Perianal disease			
Histology		*Histology*	
Deep, transmural inflammation		Mucosal inflammation	
Patchy		Continuous	
Non-caseating granulomata characteristic		Granulomata rare	
Lymphoid aggregates ++		Lymphoid aggregates rare	
Cryptitis and crypt abscesses +		Cryptitis and crypt abscesses ++	
Complications		*Complications*	
Fistula formation		No fistula	
Stricturing disease of small bowel		No small bowel involvement	
Abscess formation		Abscesses not a feature	
Vitamin B12 deficiency (ileal involvement)		Vitamin B12 deficiency rare	
Increased colonic carcinoma risk if colonic involvement; less than UC		Increased risk of colonic carcinoma	

AETIOLOGY

The cause of UC and CD remains unknown despite extensive research. Many hypotheses have been suggested including infectious agents such as measles virus and *Mycobacterium avium paratuberculosis* (MAP), environmental factors, and vascular factors. It is likely that IBD is caused by the interaction of genetic predisposition and environmental factors such as intestinal microbacteria. These interactions can probably occur at different levels, with some causing a predisposition to gut inflammation in general, some triggering UC or CD, and some determining the exact phenotype of the disease (such as disease severity and extent, and extraintestinal manifestations (**1.1**)).

Genetic factors

The possibility of a genetic component to the pathogenesis of IBD is suggested by the fact that the diseases are more common in certain populations such as Ashkenazi Jews, and through family studies, in which it is evident that CD, and to a lesser extent UC are more common in first degree relatives than in the general population. Twin studies have confirmed these observations, demonstrating over 50% concordance in monozygotic twins in CD, but lower levels in UC. The overall risk of a first degree relative developing IBD is between 5 and 20%, suggesting that genetic factors are important, but suggesting that environmental factors are also very important.

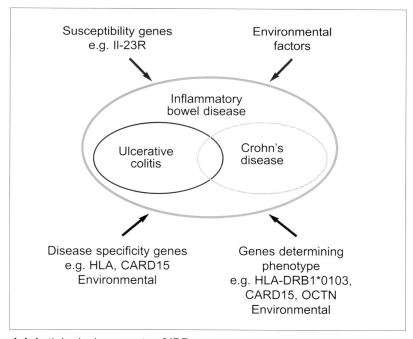

1.1 Aetiological concepts of IBD.

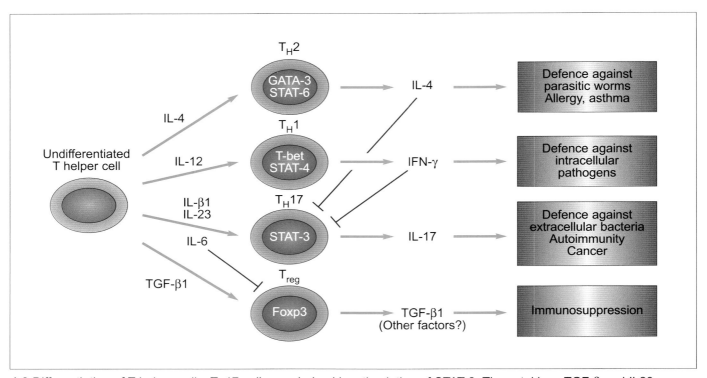

1.2 Differentiation of T helper cells. T_H17 cells are derived by stimulation of STAT-3. The cytokines TGF-β and Il-23 promote the production of these cells.

The advent of modern molecular biological techniques has allowed rapid progress to be made in the field of IBD genetics: genome-wide studies have identified a number of areas of the genome which appear to be linked to IBD, and within these a number of different genes have been identified which may play a role in triggering inflammation. These are largely related to control of the intestinal immune system and the way it reacts to the bacteria that normally exist in the gut. The most striking example of this is the CARD15 gene (NOD2) which is associated with ileal CD. This gene is part of the innate immune system, which recognizes components of bacterial cell walls (muramyl dipeptide) and triggers activation of the immune system through a series of nuclear transcription factors (most notably NF-κB). There are functional abnormalities in this process as a result of possessing CARD15 mutations, but how exactly this contributes to persistent inflammation is not yet clear. Other important genes are those of the HLA region, with the rare HLA-DRB1*0103 gene being associated with extensive and severe UC, colonic CD, and extraintestinal manifestations including large joint arthritis and uveitis. More recent studies have identified genes involved in the development and control of a novel group of T helper cells (T_H17 cells) which are characterized by the production of the cytokine Il-17. This group of cells may contribute to the pathogenesis of both forms of inflammatory bowel disease. The cytokine Il-23 has an important role in triggering undifferentiated T cells to become Il-17 producing cells, and polymorphisms in the Il-23 receptor gene have been associated with both UC and

Table 1.2 Major replicated genetic associations in IBD

Gene/region	Chromosome	Association with UC/CD	Biological function (if known)	Relative risk conferred (approx)
CARD15	16	CD – ileal disease	Intracellular receptor for muramyl dipeptide – innate immune system	2.4–30
ATG16L1	2	CD	Autophagy (programmed destruction of cellular contents)	1.5
Il23R	1	CD & UC	Receptor for Il-23 – helps differentiation of T cells to T_H17 cells	0.38 (CD) 0.73 (UC) protective
IBD5	5	CD	?	2–6
IBD3	6	CD & UC	HLA region – involved in antigen recognition and control of immune response	
IRGM		CD	Autophagy	1.4
Csome 5p13.1		CD	?	
Csome 10q21.1		CD	?	

CD. Thus it is possible that changes in the genetic control of this pathway may be important in the pathogenesis of both UC and CD. The relationships of Il-23 and T_H17 cells are illustrated in Figure **1.2**. Other genes that have been associated with IBD are involved in autophagy – the process of engulfing and destroying host cells that are no longer useful. The list of genes associated with both UC and CD grows ever larger, and now easily numbers over 40. A list of major genetic associations found in IBD is given in *Table 1.2*.

The genetic studies in IBD have clearly shown that UC and CD are not caused by abnormalities in a single gene; rather it is likely that patients have to possess a critical load of predisposing genes to develop disease (i.e. multiple genes). In addition there has to be an appropriate environmental trigger, and this seems likely to be luminal bacteria in most cases.

Environmental factors

Animal models may give an insight into the relationship between genetics and bacteria. It is possible to create models of inflammatory bowel disease by altering the genetic makeup of animals. The most well known are the HLA-B27 transgenic mouse, in which human HLA-B27 and β2-microglobulin genes are inserted, and the Il-10 knockout mouse, in which the Il-10 gene (which regulates inflammation) is deleted. In these models intestinal inflammation is not seen in animals kept in germ-free conditions, but as soon as they are reared under normal conditions the animals develop disease, demonstrating the importance of bacteria. Furthermore, different bacteria have differing abilities to cause inflammation depending on the genetic background – thus *Bacteroides* species and a cocktail of bacteria isolated from CD patients are able to cause colitis in the HLA-B27 transgenic rat, whereas *Salmonella* and *E. coli* species are less effective, and *Helicobacter hepaticus* is particularly effective at triggering inflammation in the Il-10 knockout mouse.

Table 1.3 Other theories of the aetiology of IBD

Putative causative agent	Proposed mechanism	Evidence
Mycobacterium avium sub. *paratuberculosis*	Infection with this bacteria causes granulomatous inflammation similar to Johne's disease in cattle	Isolation of MAP from some CD patients; may be a factor in some patients, unlikely to be a major cause in the majority
Measles, mumps and rubella vaccination	Combined vaccine has an effect on the overall immune system	Has now been largely disproved. In large population studies there is no increase in CD in subjects who have had the triple vaccination
Microparticles	Found in substances such as toothpastes – may excite a foreign body reaction with granulomatous inflammation	Little supporting evidence
Vascular inflammation	Inflammation of small vessels in the mesentery leading to inflammation and infarction	The anti-mesenteric nature of CD, and some evidence of vascular abnormalities. It is difficult to know whether these are primary or secondary

The challenge for investigators now is to try to unravel the complex link between the genetic background of the host and the luminal bacteria. This is particularly difficult as there are estimated to be over 400 species of intestinal bacteria, and over 40% of these are not amenable to traditional culture. New techniques such as 16S ribosomal ribonucleic acid (RNA) subunit typing may help to unpick these issues, by allowing a fuller characterization of the intestinal microbacteria. The realization of the importance of the luminal bacteria in triggering disease has also meant that much research is now being conducted into how the intestinal microbacteria may be altered to ameliorate disease, and there is currently much interest in probiotics (medications containing live bacteria to colonize the intestine) and prebiotics (foods which will favour specific bacterial species within the gut).

There have been many other theories about the pathogenesis of IBD, some of which have been highly controversial (see *Table 1.3*). These include an association between CD and the measles, mumps and rubella vaccine (MMR) and also MAP. It is clear that these agents do not cause the majority of CD, and epidemiological evidence has now made it clear that MMR is not associated with disease. MAP is clearly not the cause of most cases of CD, but there remains the possibility that it may be involved in a small proportion of cases.

Recommended reading

Cho JH. The genetics and immunopathogenesis of inflammatory bowel disease. *Nat Rev Immunol* 2008 Jun;**8**(6):458–66.

Packey CD, Sartor RB. Interplay of commensal and pathogenic bacteria, genetic mutations, and immunoregulatory defects in the pathogenesis of inflammatory bowel diseases. *J Intern Med* 2008 Jun;**263**(6):597–606.

CLINICAL PRESENTATION

Introduction

Both CD and UC follow a relapsing–remitting pattern, producing 'flares' of variable severity and duration, and the symptoms described below are frequently intermittent and self-limiting. There is therefore an inherent delay in diagnosis, as patients tend to present with a subacute history of weeks or sometimes months, with complaints usually regarded as benign, typically of infective origin, by both themselves and treating physicians.

Symptomatology in UC typically constitutes predictable complaints related to the involvement of different parts of the colon. On the other hand, the inflammatory process in CD may involve one or more segments of bowel from the mouth to the anus, either in continuity or, much more commonly, in a segmental manner, and as such, it can produce a more variable constellation of symptoms. Recent evidence suggests, however, that there may be specific patterns in the segments of bowel involved in each individual patient, as well as in the way the disease will behave in terms of its inflammatory, stricturing, and fistulizing potential. A number of attempts have been made to classify IBD based on the site of disease and its severity. Initially the Vienna classification was written for CD, and more recently the Montreal classification has aimed to establish clear and accurate clinical phenotypes of disease. This can be useful in clinical practice to help give a guide to long-term outcomes and natural history. The Vienna and Montreal classifications are shown in *Tables 1.4–1.6*. In CD the disease is classified by age at diagnosis, site of disease, and disease behaviour. In UC the disease is classified by extent and severity.

In addition, IBD can produce extraintestinal features which are either idiosyncratic due to the inflammatory response (commonly termed extraintestinal manifestations), or directly related to functional loss and malabsorption or other complications; both of these categories of symptoms will be examined separately from the luminal ones. Many of these occur at the time of first presentation and, in some cases, may be more obvious than the GI symptoms.

Table 1.4 The Vienna and Montreal classifications of CD

Vienna and Montreal classifications
Crohn's disease

	Vienna	Montreal
Age at diagnosis	A1 below 40 y	A1 below 16 y
	A2 above 40 y	A2 between 17 and 40 y
		A3 above 40 y
Location	L1 ileal	L1 ileal
	L2 colonic	L2 colonic
	L3 ileocolonic	L3 ileocolonic
	L4 upper	L4 isolated upper disease*
Behaviour	B1 non-stricturing, non-penetrating	B1 non-stricturing, non-penetrating
	B2 stricturing	B2 stricturing
	B3 penetrating	B3 penetrating
		p perianal disease modifier**

*L4 is a modifier that can be added to L1–L3 when concomitant upper gastrointestinal disease is present
** 'p' is added to B1–B3 when concomitant perianal disease is present

Adapted from Satsangi J, *et al. Gut* 2006;**55**:749–53

Table 1.5 The Montreal Classification of UC – disease extent

Disease extent

Extent	Anatomy
E1 ulcerative proctitis	Involvement limited to the rectum, i.e. proximal extent of inflammation is distal to the rectosigmoid junction
E2 left-sided UC (distal UC)	Involvement limited to the proportion of the colorectum distal to the splenic flexure
E3 extensive UC	Involvement extends proximal to the splenic flexure

Adapted from Satsangi J, *et al. Gut* 2006;**55**:749–53

Table 1.6 The Montreal Classification of UC – disease severity

Disease severity

Severity	Anatomy
S0 clinical remission	Asymptomatic
S1 mild UC	Passage of 4 or fewer stools/day (with or without blood), absence of any systemic illness, and normal imflammatory markers
S2 moderate UC	Passage of more than 4 stools per day but with minimal signs of systemic toxicity
S3 severe UC	Passage of at least 6 bloody stools daily, pulse rate of at least 90 beats per minute, temperature of at least 37.5°C, haemoglobin of less than 10.5 g/100 ml, and ESR of at least 30 mm/hr

ESR: erythrocyte sedimentation rate

Adapted from Satsangi J, *et al. Gut* 2006;**55**:749–53

Luminal symptoms of CD

Small bowel (1.3)

CD involves the small bowel in about 50% of cases. The symptomatology produced by small bowel CD can be accounted for either directly due to inflammation of the intestinal mucosa, or indirectly in terms of the manifestations of various degrees of functional loss; it mainly includes diarrhoea, abdominal pain, and weight loss. Diarrhoea is the cardinal feature of small bowel CD, and it typically persists during the night leading to sleep disturbance of variable severity. When the terminal ileum is involved to such a degree that fat and bile salt malabsorption occur, patients describe steatorrhoeic stool, which is pale in colour, stains the pan, and is difficult to flush. Other proposed mechanisms accounting for the diarrhoea in jejuno-ileitis are bacterial overgrowth, particularly proximal to stenosed segments, and a reduced capacity of the inflamed mucosa to absorb water, which is more significant pathophysiologically in large bowel CD. Abdominal pain may be due to the inflamed segments or due to the effects of bowel wall oedema and subsequently stricturing. When strictures are responsible for the abdominal pain it usually occurs within 1 or 2 hours after food, and it is more prominent following consumption of high-fibre diets. Depending on severity, strictures can be associated with various degrees of post-prandial abdominal distention and vomiting. Weight loss, which is typically modest, is also multifactorial, and it can be accounted for by the catabolic state of the inflammatory response, the malabsorption, and the food avoidance resulting from the post-prandial exacerbation of symptoms.

Large bowel (1.4)

Large bowel CD occurs either in isolation or in combination with terminal ileal disease, when the caecum and ascending colon are preferentially involved. Diarrhoea is again a prominent feature and may be attributed to the reduced capacity of the inflamed mucosa to resorb water as well as to alterations in transit times. Excessive inflammation results in variable amounts of rectal bleeding associated with the diarrhoea, which is more pronounced when distal segments are involved. In addition, patients with rectal inflammation frequently present with urgency and incontinence as the capacity of the inflamed rectum is reduced. This is often a debilitating symptom severely affecting quality of life. Furthermore, with more distal involvement patients frequently describe a mucoid appearance of the stool, or even the sole passage of blood and/or mucus independent of the diarrhoea.

Pain produced by large bowel inflammation is usually crampy in character, preceding and relieved by defecation. As the inflammation in CD is typically transmural, serosal wall abscesses may form, resulting in more severe and persisting pain, localized peritonitis, and a septic state.

Fistulae and perianal involvement

Fistula formation is one of the most distressing complications in CD, occurring in approximately one-third of patients. In fistulizing forms of the condition, fistulae may form between segments of the bowel, presenting with high-output diarrhoea and pain, in addition to the effects of the usually profound electrolyte depletion. Occasionally fistulae may form between the small intestine and the bladder or the female reproductive organs, producing the corresponding local symptoms of recurrent urinary tract infection, pneumaturia or faecuria, as well as abnormal vaginal discharges.

Perianal involvement has a varying reported prevalence according to the distribution of the luminal pathology, ranging from >90% of patients with Crohn's colitis with rectal involvement to 12% of patients with isolated small bowel disease. Common findings include skin tags and haemorrhoids, anal fissures which are frequently painless, perianal fistulae and abscesses, anal canal stenosis and, rarely, anal cancer. They contribute significantly to morbidity, and together with fistulae described above they constitute the most persistent manifestations of CD, commonly requiring protracted medical and surgical management.

Oesophagus–stomach

The upper GI tract is the least commonly involved segment. When the oesophagus is involved, odynophagia and dysphagia are the cardinal symptoms. In cases of gastric involvement, patients complain of nausea, vomiting, and epigastric pain.

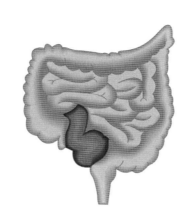

Symptoms

Diarrhoea

Abdominal pain

Weight loss

Symptoms of
malabsorption

1.3 Symptoms of small bowel CD.

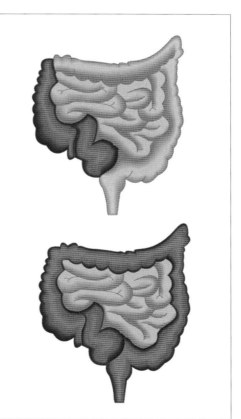

A combination of

Diarrhoea

Abdominal pain

Weight loss

Symptoms of
malabsorption

and

Rectal bleeding

Urgency
(according to
degree of large
bowel involvement)

1.4 Symptoms of large bowel (ileocolonic) CD.

Luminal symptoms of UC

Proctitis (1.5)

Patients with proctitis usually complain of the passage of fresh blood, or blood-stained mucus, which is either mixed with stool or streaked onto its surface. Tenesmus and urgency are also prominent features, with episodes of incontinence being not uncommon. In addition, many patients may actually complain of constipation, frequently confirmed on imaging, which has been attributed to slower whole colon transit times in the presence of distal constipation.

Left-sided and extensive disease (1.6)

As the disease extends beyond the rectosigmoid, episodes of bloody diarrhoea, frequently containing pus, are the predominant feature. As in CD, multiple nocturnal episodes of diarrhoea frequently lead to sleep disturbance. Abdominal pain of variable severity is also a feature of more extensive colitis, both in the form of lower abdominal discomfort as well as central abdominal cramping.

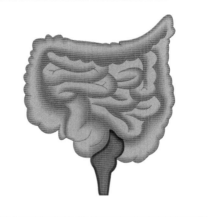

Symptoms

Fresh mucosal bleeding (with mucus)

Tenesmus

Urgency/incontinence

1.5 Symptoms of proctitis.

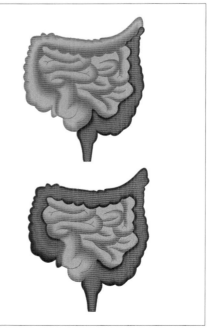

Symptoms

Variable amounts of bloody diarrhoea (related to extent of disease and severity of inflammation)

Crampy, lower abdominal pain

1.6 Symptoms of left-sided and extensive disease.

Extraintestinal manifestations

The life-time risk for the development of extraintestinal manifestations (EIMs) in both UC and CD is around 25–30%, and they occasionally precede or predominate over the GI symptoms. Thus, in patients presenting with features of possible EIMs of a GI condition, a careful GI history should be obtained at the onset, in an attempt to establish if IBD is a likely underlying diagnosis.

Cutaneous manifestations

Up to 10% of patients with IBD describe cutaneous symptoms, most commonly erythema nodosum, pyoderma gangrenosum, and oral manifestations. Erythema nodosum is characterized by sudden-onset painful bilateral nodules of average diameter around 2 cm. They commonly occur on the shins but have also been described on the calves, face, and trunk. It is more common in UC, and it usually mirrors the activity of the luminal disease. Pyoderma gangrenosum has been described in 0.5–20% and 1–10% of patients with CD and UC, respectively. Pain typically precedes the development of pustules and the rapid formation of a necrotic ulcer with bluish borders. Like erythema nodosum, the overwhelming majority occurs on the lower legs. Oral manifestations of IBD include aphthous ulceration, which occur in about 10% of patients, and may constitute the presenting complaint. Painful mucosal cobblestoning and pyostomatitis vegetans have also been described.

Musculoskeletal manifestations

Central arthropathies related to IBD include a range of syndromes. Asymptomatic sacraliitis detected by radiological evidence only has an estimated prevalence of up to 50%. At the other end of the spectrum, full-blown ankylosing spondylitis occurs in approximately 5% of patients. Inflammatory back pain characteristically is low back pain at night or at rest, and improving with movement, and occurs in up to 30% of patients with CD. It typically radiates to the buttocks, is associated with morning stiffness for more than 30 minutes, and responds well to nonsteroidal anti-inflammatory medication. It is often a challenge to distinguish this pain from mechanical low back pain, which is very common.

Peripheral arthropathies occur in 5–20% of patients with IBD and they are subcategorized into Type I (pauciarticular, large joints, fewer than 5 joints involved with evidence of swelling and effusion, mainly asymmetrical) and Type II (polyarticular, with 5 or more joints involved with evidence of swelling and effusion, mainly symmetrical). Both types occur significantly more commonly in women. In 25–30% of large joint arthritis (Type I), the arthritis is one of the presenting features of the IBD. Clinically, it is identical to a post-enteric infection reactive arthritis. Thus, in patients who present with large joint arthritis in combination with intestinal symptoms, a rectal biopsy looking for signs of chronic inflammation is often helpful. If the GI symptoms persist, then a colonoscopy is mandatory.

Ocular manifestations

Ocular manifestations of IBD occur in less than 10% of patients but contribute significantly to overall morbidity in those affected. Episcleritis is the commonest complication and typically flares during increases in IBD activity, and it should be suspected in patients presenting with acute unilateral or bilateral redness, irritation, and burning. When photophobia and reduction of visual acuity are superimposed on the above symptoms, then scleritis or uveitis should be suspected, prompting an urgent ophthalmological referral.

Hepato-biliary manifestations

Primary sclerosing cholangitis is the main hepato-biliary manifestation of IBD, with a prevalence of up to 3% of cases. Although usually detected in the asymptomatic phase, patients may present with symptoms of biliary stasis, such as jaundice and pruritus, and, in late cases, biliary sepsis may ensue.

Symptoms related to complications

Manifestations of malabsorption

CD affecting the small bowel can result in malabsorption and nutritional deficiencies, which produce a wide symptomatology (outlined in *Table 1.7*).

Thromboembolic events

IBD has been increasingly recognized as an independent risk factor for the development of venous thromboembolism (VTE). A high clinical suspicion should therefore be maintained both for symptoms at common sites such as leg swelling, pleuritic chest pain, and shortness of breath as well as at rarer locations, e.g. arm swelling in axillary/subclavian thromboses and neurological symptoms in cerebral venous sinus thromboses.

Recommended reading

American Gastroenterological Association medical position statement: Peri-anal Crohn's disease. *Gastroenterology* 2003;**125**:1503–7.

DeVos M. Review article: Joint involvement in inflammatory bowel disease. *Aliment Pharmacol Ther* 2004;**20**(suppl. 4):36–42.

Mintz R, *et al*. Ocular manifestations of inflammatory bowel disease. *Inflamm Bowel Dis* 2004 Mar;**10**(2):135–9. Review.

Orchard TR, *et al*. Peripheral arthropathies in inflammatory bowel disease: their articular distribution and natural history. *Gut* 1998;**42**;387–91.

Trost LB, *et al*. Important cutaneous manifestations of inflammatory bowel disease. *Post-grad Med J* 2005;**81**:580–5.

Table 1.7 Symptoms of malabsorption and nutritional deficiencies

Nutrient	Symptoms of deficiency/excess
Albumin	Generalized dependent oedema, cardiac failure, altered handling of several drugs
Calcium	Neuromuscular: perioral and peripheral tingling, cramps/tetany, bronchospasm Neurological: irritability, depression, behavioural changes, seizures Cardiac: shortness of breath, congestive cardiac failure Cutaneous: coarse hair, brittle nails, psoriasis, dry skin
Magnesium	Weakness, muscle cramping, palpitations
Oxalate	Renal colic, gross haematuria
Niacin	Pellagra-like symptoms
B12	Symptoms of anaemia, peripheral neuropathy

Chapter 2

Investigations at diagnosis

Introduction

The diagnosis of IBD is confirmed by clinical evaluation and a combination of laboratory, endoscopic, radiological, and histological investigations. Wherever possible a histological diagnosis is obtained, either by biopsy at endoscopy or from operative specimens. However, it may not always be possible to obtain tissue for histology, particularly in cases of isolated small bowel CD, where the diagnosis may rest on the history and appropriate radiological appearances.

Laboratory investigations

A number of baseline laboratory investigations should be undertaken, in terms of both blood and faecal samples.

Full blood count

Anaemia may result from acute/chronic blood loss, malabsorption (iron, folate, and vitamin B12) or anaemia of chronic disease. Vitamin B12 deficiency is most common in patients with terminal ileal CD, and the finding of a low B12 level should trigger investigation of the terminal ileum. The platelet count may be elevated in acute inflammation and a modestly raised white blood cell (WBC) count is observed in active colitis. A marked elevation in WBC, with a neutrophilia, should raise suspicion of an acute infection or abscess formation.

Biochemistry

Potassium and magnesium stores become depleted in patients with chronic diarrhoea. In patients with extensive CD malabsorption may be a problem, leading to decreased levels of calcium, and in both IBDs persistent inflammation may lead to decreased albumin levels. As there is a known association between IBD and primary sclerosing cholangitis (PSC), liver function tests should be checked. The first sign of PSC associated with IBD may be an isolated elevation of alkaline phosphatase, progressing to a more general obstructive picture in the liver function tests.

Inflammatory markers

C-reactive protein (CRP) and erythrocyte sedimentation rate (ESR) are markers of acute inflammation and will be raised in both infections and inflammation of the bowel. However, it should be noted that in both UC and CD there is a subgroup of patients in whom systemic inflammatory markers such as ESR and CRP remain normal. If levels are elevated when the disease is active, measurement of ESR and CRP is an effective way to monitor inflammatory activity.

Stool microscopy, culture, and sensitivity (MC&S)

MC&S will help to exclude an infective cause for diarrhoea. Three samples should be sent for full MC&S.

Clostridium difficile

Clostridium difficile is becoming more common, particularly following recent antibiotic administration, and a test for *Clostridium difficile* toxin (CDT) should be routinely requested in patients with acute diarrhoea. Further characterization by ribotyping can be considered if there is doubt about the diagnosis. Up to 10–15% of hospitalized patients with IBD may have co-existing *C. difficile* infection, and for this reason any hospitalized patients with a flare of their colitis should have a CDT test requested. However patients may also develop *C. difficile* in the community and so it should also be tested for in patients who present to the outpatient department. It is important to note that a proportion of patients with *C. difficile*-associated diarrhoea do not test positive for the toxin, and so if there is a preceding history of antibiotic therapy and a high index of suspicion then per testing and possibly endoscopy and biopsy should be undertaken.

Stool tests

Additional stool tests may be needed for patients who have travelled abroad (stool ova and parasite studies). These require analysis of fresh stool samples. Amoebiasis can be particularly difficult to identify in the stool so further serological testing may be required if there is a high level of suspicion.

Faecal calprotectin

Calprotectin is a protein released by neutrophils, and so measurement of faecal calprotectin can be a good marker of acute inflammation. It does not help determine whether the cause of the inflammation is infective, due to IBD, or due to other causes such as nonsteroidal anti-inflammatory drugs (NSAIDs), but can help to distinguish functional bowel symptoms. It can be used to monitor inflammatory activity in patients in whom the diagnosis of IBD is established.

Endoscopy

Endoscopy is now the gold standard for the diagnosis of IBD, as it allows direct visualization of the mucosa and offers the opportunity to take biopsies for histological examination. Endoscopy is required in virtually all patients with IBD. The exact procedure undertaken will depend upon the nature of the disease and its extent.

Sigmoidoscopy

Rigid sigmoidoscopy

This may be undertaken in the setting of the outpatient clinic, without any bowel preparation. In UC, where the rectum is nearly always affected, it allows a diagnosis to be made quickly, although it will not allow an estimation of extent unless the disease is confined to the rectum only, and there is normal mucosa visible above the affected segment. In patients in whom a diagnosis of UC has been established it can be used to monitor disease activity. It is important to remember that if the patient is taking topical therapy, the lower colon may look relatively unaffected, whereas there may be more significant inflammation more proximally. In CD, where the rectum is often spared, rigid sigmoidoscopy is a less effective tool for monitoring disease activity, unless there is a well established history of rectal disease.

Flexible sigmoidoscopy

This may be performed unprepared or with bowel preparation with a phosphate enema or laxative. It does not normally require sedation, and is relatively quick. It can be used to monitor patients with left-sided UC, and to investigate patients in whom bright red rectal bleeding is a problem. It can also be performed in the acute setting on patients admitted with acute severe colitis. In this setting no bowel preparation is used, and biopsies are taken to assess disease activity and to exclude superimposed infection, particularly due to *C. difficile* and cytomegalovirus (CMV).

Ileocolonoscopy

This is the investigation of choice for patients with IBD. It allows visualization of the colon and also the terminal ileum in the majority of cases. This may be very important in determining whether a patient has UC or CD. In order to be effective the bowel should be prepared over the preceding days by a low-fibre diet and purgative laxatives such as sodium picophosphate to allow close inspection of the mucosa. It allows the determination of disease extent and activity, both on endoscopic appearance, and also by histological appearance. It is the favoured form of investigation for surveillance for colorectal cancer in IBD patients. In these circumstances the sensitivity of the examination is enhanced by the use of chromoendoscopy, where dyes such as indigo-carmine are sprayed onto the mucosa to highlight irregularities that should be biopsied.

Appearances at endoscopy

Visualizing the colonic mucosa helps confirm the presence of inflammation or a source of bleeding (such as haemorrhoids) within the reach of the scope and allows biopsies to be taken for histological evaluation.

Typical features of UC include loss of the vascular pattern with oedema, granularity, ulceration, and contact bleeding of the mucosa (**2.1–2.5**). In patients with long-standing colitis where there has been substantial activity there may be the appearance of pseudopolyps, due to polypoid regeneration after inflammation (**2.6**). These polyps are not adenomatous, or neoplastic as such, but indicate a high degree of previous inflammatory activity.

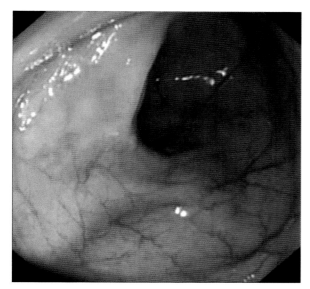

2.1 Normal colonic mucosa in the sigmoid colon.

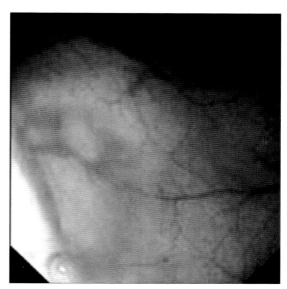

2.2 Normal vascular pattern in the colon showing clear delineation of the blood vessels.

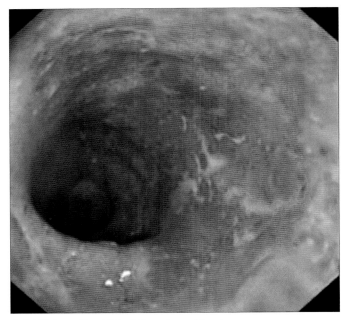

2.3 Mildy active UC of the sigmoid colon.

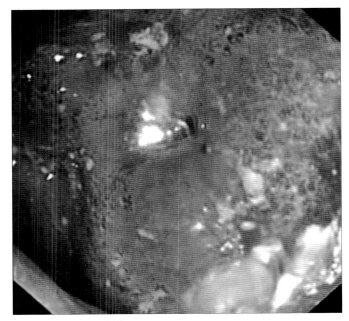

2.4 Mildy active UC.

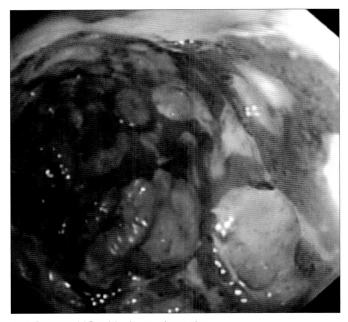

2.5 Severe UC with deep ulceration.

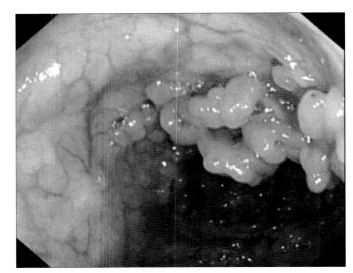

2.6 Pseudopolyps in UC.

CD has a macroscopic appearance of focal, asymmetric inflammation of the colonic mucosa with or without ulceration in the terminal ileum. The ulcers vary from small aphthoid ulcers to deep serpiginous ulcers (**2.7**). There may also be endoscopic appearances of cobblestoning, where the ulcers lead to the appearance of cobbles with deep crevices between them.

In contrast to colitis secondary to IBD, *Clostridium difficile* has a typical appearance of raised yellow-white plaques termed pseudomembranes (**2.8**).

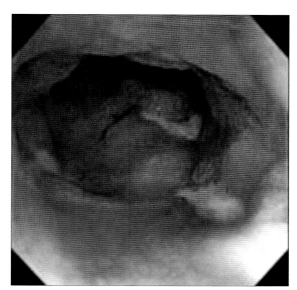

2.7 Ulceration of the terminal ileum in CD.

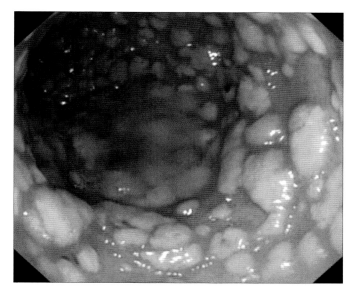

2.8 Pseudomembranes secondary to *C. difficile* colitis.

Upper GI endoscopy (oesophago-gastro-duodenoscopy (OGD))

CD can affect the upper GI tract in 5–10% of patients; therefore, in patients with upper GI symptoms, an OGD should be requested to check for aphthous ulceration.

Capsule endoscopy

More recently, wireless capsule endoscopy, used most often to investigate the source of GI bleeding, has been found useful in diagnosing mucosal lesions in CD. It is most useful in the diagnosis of CD in patients with occult gastrointestinal bleeding of unknown cause, where the lesions of CD may be demonstrated in the small bowel. It may also be used to assess diffuse small bowel disease, where it may be more sensitive than contrast studies. However,

patients must be examined carefully to determine that there are no strictures or bowel obstructions before the capsule can be used. This should ideally be done by a contrast study prior to the capsule endoscopy. The technique is performed by having the patient swallow an encapsulated video camera that transmits images to a receiver which is strapped to the patient's belt. A number of external pads are used to detect the position of the capsule within the body in real time to allow localization of any lesions that are found on the video. The capsule is passed in the faeces, and the video is then viewed to identify any lesions. Complications that may occur include nonretrieval of the capsule, intestinal obstruction, and rarely intestinal perforation. The appearance of CD as seen at capsule endoscopy is shown in Figure **2.9**.

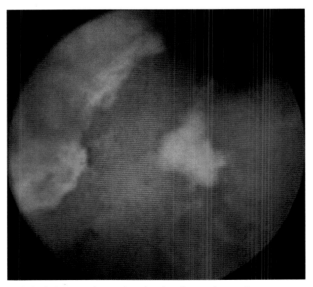

2.9 Aphthous ulceration in the ileum in early CD seen at capsule endoscopy.

Radiology

With the advent of more advanced endoscopy the requirement for radiographic examinations has decreased, but radiographs still have an important role to play in the investigation of IBD.

Abdominal X-ray

A plain abdominal radiograph is not required in every patient presenting to the outpatient department, as it is not a particularly effective diagnostic tool. Patients may have a normal X-ray or it may show an empty colon up to the extent of the disease. A plain abdominal X-ray (AXR) is, however, essential in the initial assessment of patients with suspected severe IBD, when colonic oedema giving a 'thumb printing' appearance or mucosal islands may be seen on AXR (**2.10**). These are the appearances of islands of intact mucosa in severe inflammation, and indicate a high likelihood of imminent perforation.

AXR will help to assess disease extent in UC and identify proximal constipation in patients with left-sided colitis. Most importantly, the plain AXR can detect a toxic megacolon (a long continuous segment of air-filled colon with dilatation >6 cm; **2.11**), which can be seen in acute severe colitis and requires urgent surgical referral.

Repeat radiographs at 24-hour intervals to monitor the course of dilatation and to assess the need for emergency colectomy are essential in the acute stages of severe colitis.

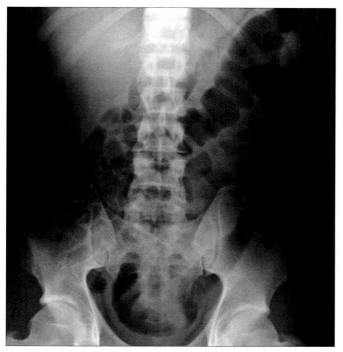

2.10 AXR of patient with acute UC showing a featureless left colon with an oedematous wall demonstrating 'thumb printing'.

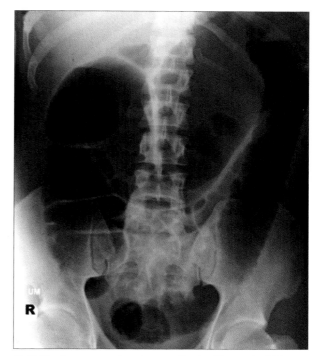

2.11 Toxic megacolon in a patient with acute UC.

Double contrast barium enema

This is usually inferior to colonoscopy as an examination of the colon, and is less commonly used than previously because it does not allow mucosal biopsy and may underestimate the extent of disease. Loss of haustrations and destruction of the mucosal pattern indicate colitis in this examination. Barium enema is contraindicated in patients with moderate-to-severe colitis because it risks perforation or precipitation of a toxic megacolon.

Small bowel imaging

If CD is suspected then further radiological tests should be requested to visualize the small bowel.

Barium follow through or small bowel enteroclysis (small bowel enema) are X-ray contrast studies of the small intestine. Small bowel enteroclysis, where barium is given via intubation of the small bowel through a nasojejenal tube, is probably a better examination because the contrast is delivered directly to the small bowel. This allows the contrast to be injected with a higher pressure, and means that contrast does not remain in the stomach, obscuring views of the small bowel. However, small bowel follow-through examinations, where the contrast is ingested orally, are easier to perform, and may be more readily available. There is considerable operator variability in both the performance and interpretation of these tests; an experienced GI radiologist is required to use them to their full potential.

In CD, areas of segmental narrowing with loss of normal mucosa, fistula formation, and the string sign (a narrow band of barium flowing through an inflamed or scarred area) in the terminal ileum may be observed (**2.12**). In areas of inflammation and ulceration characteristic 'rose thorn' ulcers may be observed as inflamed loops of bowel, which are spread apart more than usual.

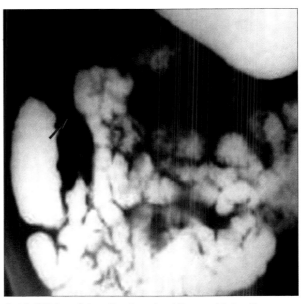

2.12 CD involving the terminal ileum. Note: the string sign indicated by the arrow.

CT scanning

CT scanning may be used to assess IBD. It is helpful if perforation is suspected, and may allow an estimation of disease extent, although it is not the most effective modality for doing this. It has a particular role in delineating the anatomy of complex inflammatory masses in CD, where there may be multiple loops of bowel which are adherent, and which may contain multiple strictures. In addition, it is the investigation of choice if an abscess or collection is suspected.

White cell scanning

This is a safe and noninvasive investigation. It lacks specificity and is therefore not routinely used for diagnosis or initial assessment of IBD. It is particularly useful in investigating atypical symptoms, to determine whether there is any localization of white cells to the bowel, which would indicate active inflammation. The technique is performed by radio-labelling a sample of the patient's own white cells with either indium[111] or technetium[99]. The latter probably provides slightly better resolution. The patient is then visualized using a gamma camera to identify the areas where the white cells localize, indicating probable areas of inflammation.

Ultrasound

In skilled hands ultrasound is a sensitive and noninvasive way of identifying thickened small bowel loops in CD and may identify abscesses and fistulae in the peritoneum. It is, however, very operator dependent.

Magnetic resonance imaging (MRI)

MRI is a noninvasive, nonionizing radiation technique and is especially helpful in identifying precise localization of the disease. It is the investigation of choice for identifying the anatomy of fistulizing CD, particularly in the pelvis and perineum, and may be used to assess response to therapy. MRI enteroclysis is also becoming more widely available as an alternative to traditional methods of imaging the small bowel in the diagnosis and assessment of CD. A case of small bowel CD on MRI scanning is illustrated in Figure **2.13**.

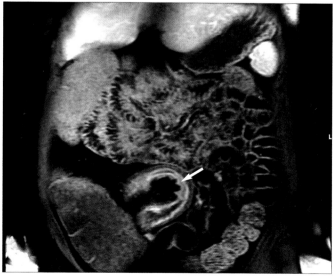

2.13 An MRI scan of the small bowel demonstrating a segment of terminal ileal CD, with wall thickening, and enhancement with significant luminal narrowing.

Table 2.1 Investigations used in IBD

Situation	Rigid Σ	Flex Σ	Colonoscopy	Capsule endoscopy	Ba FT/ enteroclysis	CT scan	MRI/MRI enteroclysis (e)	WCC scan	US
Initial diagnosis UC	√	√	√						
Initial diagnosis CD			√	√	√		√ (e)		√
Initial assessment UC		√	√						
Initial assessment CD			√	√	√	√	√ (e)		
Assessment of activity UC	√	√	√						
Assessment of activity CD			√					√	
Fistulae					√	√	√		
Strictures			√		√		√		
Abscesses						√	√	√	√

Histopathology

Histopathology is a vital part of the diagnosis of IBD and in the assessment of its activity. It is covered in more detail in the next chapter. However, in UC the inflammation is limited to the mucosa which almost always involves the rectum and is continuous. UC only involves the colon and the remainder of the GI tract is not inflamed, although rarely 'backwash' ileitis may be seen associated with severe extensive UC. Biopsy specimens demonstrate neutrophilic infiltrate along with crypt abscesses and crypt distortion. Granulomas do not generally occur in UC. In CD the entire intestinal wall is involved, not just the mucosa as in UC. Biopsy specimens may demonstrate granulomas, which are helpful for making the diagnosis but are not essential. Laparoscopy may be necessary in selected patients, especially where the differential diagnosis of intestinal tuberculosis is being considered.

A summary of the types of investigation used in IBD in differing circumstances is found in *Table 2.1*.

Recommended reading

Stange EF, Travis SPL, Vermeire S, *et al.* European consensus on the diagnosis and management of Crohn's disease: definitions and diagnosis. *Gut* 2006;55:1–15.

Stange EF, Travis SPL, Vermeire S, *et al.* European evidence-based consensus on the diagnosis and management of ulcerative colitis: definitions and diagnosis. *J Crohn's Colitis* 2008;2:1–23.

Chapter 3

Pathology of inflammatory bowel disease

Introduction

The role of the pathologist in dealing with cases of IBD is to help in making the diagnosis, assessing its severity, and identifying its complications. Often the first challenge is to distinguish IBD from other causes of colitis (especially self-limiting colitis (infectious)) and only then to contribute to making the specific diagnosis of CD or UC. On the initial biopsy cases of UC usually already show evidence of chronicity (with architectural distortion), whereas this is less commonly the case with CD and seen only rarely in infectious colitis. The inflammation in UC is microscopically and macroscopically diffuse while in both CD and infection it is frequently focal. Although granulomas are characteristic of CD, they are frequently not seen in otherwise typical cases and may be present in typical cases of UC when they are in association with ruptured crypts. They may also be seen in association with an infective colitis.

The main differential diagnoses to be considered are as follows:

Differential diagnosis of UC
- CD/indeterminate colitis (IBD, unclassified (IBDU)).
- Acute self-limiting (infectious) colitis.
- Drug-induced colitis.
- Ischaemic colitis.
- Diverticular disease.
- Eosinophilic colitis.

Differential diagnosis of CD
- UC.
- Acute self-limiting (infectious) colitis.
- Drug-induced colitis.
- Diversion colitis.
- Ischaemic colitis.
- Diverticular disease.
- Tuberculosis and other infections.
- Microscopic colitis.

Three of the most important differential diagnoses to consider are acute self-limiting (infectious) colitis, drug-induced colitis, and diverticular disease. This is because they may closely mimic IBD and are all relatively common conditions. The differential diagnostic features are summarized below:

Acute self-limiting (infectious) colitis
- Neutrophils in the lamina propria and surface epithelium.
- No basal plasmacytosis.
- No crypt distortion.

Drug-induced colitis
- Increased apoptosis of the surface epithelium.
- Increased numbers of eosinophils and the presence of pigmented macrophages in the superficial lamina propria.

Diverticular disease
- May see: loss of plasma cell gradient, crypt inflammation, granulomas, and architectural distortion.
- Colitis only present in areas of diverticula (usually the sigmoid).

Microscopic colitis (3.1)
- Lymphocytic colitis: increased numbers of intraepithelial lymphocytes (more than 20/100 epithelial cells) and/or
- Collagenous colitis: increased thickness of the sub-epidermal collagen plate (more than 10 micrometer).

Pathology of CD

One of the characteristics of CD is that it might involve any part of the GI tract. Its key pathological features are that the inflammation is focal, transmural, and there may be associated granulomas. It should be noted that CD may be diagnosed histologically in macroscopically normal mucosa. In other words, it is a cause of a 'microscopic' colitis (along with lymphocytic and collagenous colitis).

The macroscopic appearance of CD includes:
- Granular serosa.
- Fat wrapping.
- Oedematous/fibrotic wall.
- Strictures.
- Skip lesions (3.2).
- Aphthous ulcers, serpiginous ulcers, cobblestone mucosa.
- Fissures, fistulae, or sinuses (3.3).
- Rectal sparing with mainly right-sided involvement.

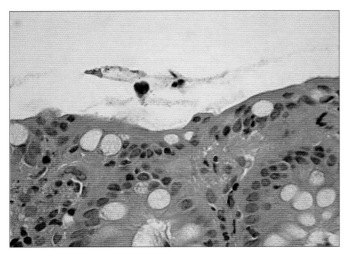

3.1 Lymphocytic colitis with an increased number of lymphocytes.

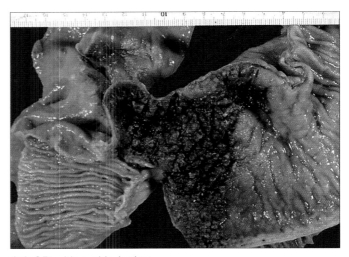

3.2 CD with a skip lesion.

The microscopic appearance of CD includes:

- Ulceration which characteristically extends deep into the bowel wall.
- Transmural inflammation with lymphoid aggregates.
- Granulomas in up to two-thirds of cases, usually near vessels (**3.4**).
- Cryptitis/crypt abscess formation (**3.5**).
- Microscopic skip lesions with relative preservation of crypt architecture (**3.6**).

- Paneth cell and pyloric gland metaplasia.
- Goblet cells present.
- Submucosal oedema.
- Mural fibrosis.
- Serosal inflammation.
- Neuronal hyperplasia.

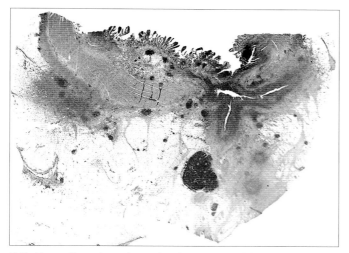

3.3 Deep fissuring ulceration in a case of CD.

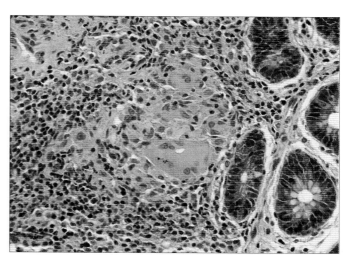

3.4 Epithelioid granulomas are a characteristic feature of CD.

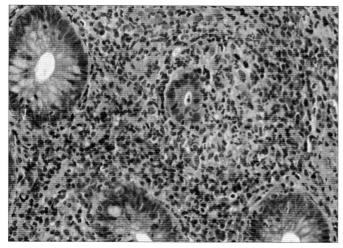

3.5 CD with crypt rupture.

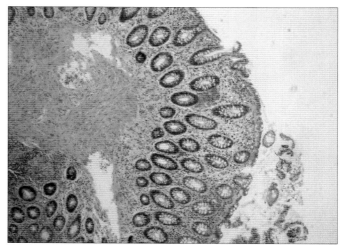

3.6 In contrast to UC, crypt architecture is relatively preserved in CD.

The diagnostic features of CD include:

- Transmural lymphoid aggregates (in areas not deeply ulcerated).
- Granulomas (not associated with ruptured glands).
- Small bowel involvement.

The importance of making a definite diagnosis of CD is that it determines the most appropriate medical and surgical treatment.

The complications of CD can be divided into intestinal and extraintestinal.

Intestinal complications of CD include:

- Strictures: especially in the terminal ileum.
- Fistulae: to loops of bowel, bladder, vagina, and perianal skin.
- Malabsorption: generalized, protein losing enteropathy, Vitamin B12 deficiency, bile salt malabsorption.
- Toxic megacolon (less common than in UC).
- Carcinoma.
- Discontinuous inflammation at sites in the gut distant from colon or small bowel (**3.7**).

Extraintestinal symptoms of CD include:

- Joints: migratory polyarthritis, sacroiliitis, ankylosing spondylitis.
- Skin: erythema nodosum, pyoderma gangrenosum, clubbing of fingers.
- Liver: PSC, pericholangitis.
- Eye: uveitis.
- Renal: secondary to periureteral fibrosis.

CD-associated carcinoma of the colon is preceded by the same changes seen in UC (see below).

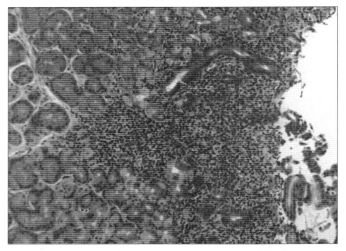

3.7 Focal gastric inflammation representing CD distant from colon or ileum.

Pathology of UC

Except in the case of 'backwash ileitis' (see below), UC is a continuous disease, starting in the rectum, which is confined to the large bowel. The inflammation is limited to the mucosa except in very active cases.

The macroscopic appearance of UC (3.8) typically include:

- Diffuse disease extends from the rectum proximally, and is confined to the large bowel.
- Disease is more active distally.
- Usually no deep fissuring ulceration, fistulae, or sinuses occur.
- No strictures.
- No bowel wall thickening.
- No serosal involvement.
- Early disease: haemorrhagic, granular, friable mucosa.
- Late disease: linear ulceration, pseudopolyps, and atrophic mucosa.

Some cases of UC may show features more typical of CD, including:

- Discontinuous or patchy disease (see below).
- Backwash ileitis (see below).
- Extracolonic inflammation.
- Granulomatous inflammation in response to ruptured crypts.
- Aphthous ulcers.
- Transmural inflammation.

Discontinuous or patchy disease in UC

- Following drug treatment (may even have normal biopsies).
- Focal disease seen in the ascending colon, caecum, and/or appendix (in patients with left-sided disease).
- Initial presentation in children.
- ?Upper GI involvement.

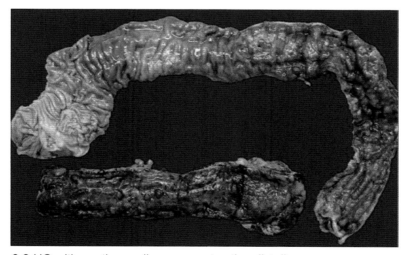

3.8 UC with continous disease most active distally.

'Backwash ileitis' in UC (approximately 20% of cases)

- Involved segment 1–2 cm long.
- Usually seen in association with caecal disease.
- Usually the changes seen are mild and include villous atrophy, increased inflammation, and scattered crypt abscesses.
- No evidence of chronicity.
- Not associated with an increased rate of ileo-anal pouch complications.

The microscopic appearance in UC includes:

- Superficial inflammation (except in severe cases).
- **Active changes** – *more marked distally*:
- loss of inflammatory cell gradient in lamina propria with basal plasmacytosis;
- cryptitis/crypt abscesses (**3.9, 3.10**);
- mucin depletion;
- ulceration.

- **Chronic changes** (*N.B. usually present even in recently diagnosed cases*):
- crypt architectural distortion (**3.11, 3.12**);
- regenerative epithelial changes;
- Paneth cell metaplasia (*normally present on the right side of the large bowel*) (**3.13**);
- endocrine cell hyperplasia;
- pseudopolyps.

Diagnostic features of UC include:

- Rectal involvement with continuous proximal involvement (limited to the colon).
- No skip lesions.
- No granulomas.
- No transmural inflammation.
- No deep fissures/sinuses.

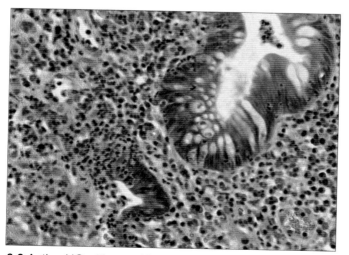

3.9 Active UC with cryptitis.

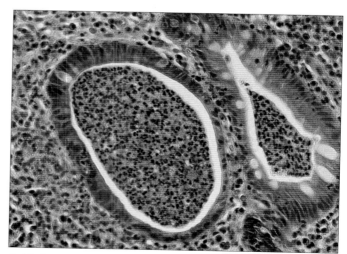

3.10 Crypt inflammation, with crypt abscess formation, is seen in active UC.

3.11 Histology in UC.

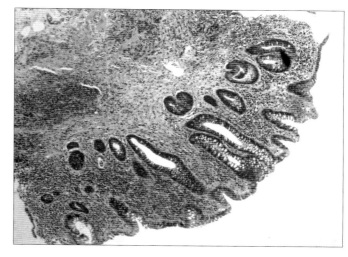

3.12 Inactive UC, crypt architectural disortion, no active inflammation.

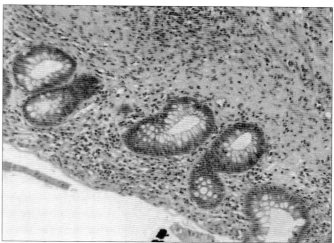

3.13 Paneth cell metaplasia in a case of UC which indicates chronic damage.

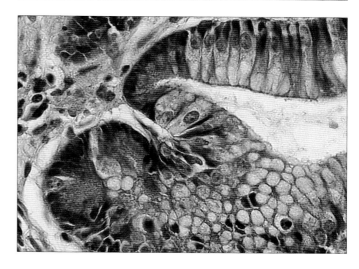

Extraintestinal manifestations of UC include:
- Joints: migratory polyarthritis, sacroiliitis, ankylosing spondylitis.
- Skin: pyoderma gangrenosum, erythema nodosum, clubbing of fingers.
- Liver: PSC, pericholangitis, cholangiocarcinoma.
- Eye: uveitis.

Complications of UC include:
- CMV infection in 25% (often detectable only by immunohistochemistry) (**3.14**).
- Perforation.
- Toxic megacolon.
- Iliac vein thrombosis.
- Carcinoma, lymphoma.

Paediatric ulcerative colitis is more likely to:
- Be patchy.
- Show histological evidence of chronicity.
- Show rectal sparing.
- Have an initial pancolitis.

Malignancy in IBD

The detection of IBD-associated dysplasia can be demanding for the pathologist. It may be seen in flat mucosa or as a mass lesion (a dysplasia-associated lesion/mass – DALM). In the latter case it needs to be distinguished from a sporadic adenoma. The three features which are most valuable for making this distinction are that the polyps are located outside of current active disease, that they have histological features of sporadic adenoma, and that there is an uneventful course following polypectomy. Biopsies from mucosa around the base of the polyp may also be helpful as DALMs may be associated with more widespread dysplasia. Immunohistochemistry has a limited role in this differential diagnosis. As is the general rule with the assessment of dysplasia in the GI tract, the biopsies should be reviewed by two histopathologists.

Dysplasia in IBD
- Usually detected by surveillance colonoscopy with biopsy.
- Multiple biopsies are recommended for diagnosis of flat lesions.
- Precedes carcinoma in almost all cases.
- Incidence of dysplasia is 2% after 10 years of UC, 18% after 30 years of UC.
- Dysplasia is rare (less than 3%) in retained rectal segment after anastomosis.

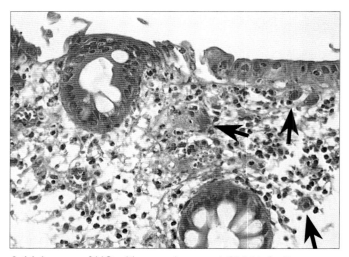

3.14 A case of UC with superimposed CMV infection.

The microscopic appearance of dysplasia (3.15) includes:

- **Low-grade dysplasia**: basally oriented nuclei; mild nuclear enlargement, nuclear crowding, and hyperchromasia; decreased intracellular mucin.
- **High-grade dysplasia**:
  - prominent nuclear stratification; more marked hyperchromasia and pleomorphism;
  - may have marked architectural distortion with a villous or nodular growth pattern.
- **Indefinite for dysplasia:** epithelial changes in a background of active inflammation with regeneration.

UC-associated carcinoma

- 10–20% are multiple (especially in younger individuals).
- Usually arise from flat mucosa.
- Often poorly differentiated/mucinous carcinomas.
- Often advanced stage.

Pathological changes seen after surgery for IBD

Patients with UC and CD may come to surgery. Because of the high risk of pouch complications in CD, all the diagnostic information, including the histology, should be reviewed before a decision to operate is taken. The operative specimen should, of course, be carefully reviewed. There are a significant number of cases in which a definite diagnosis of either CD or UC cannot be made. Some of these cases fall into one of the following three groups:

1 Patchy disease in UC (see above).
2 Anal lesions or 'backwash' ileitis and appendicitis (in continuity with severe colitis) in UC.
3 Fulminant UC (in which there may be superficial fissuring, transmural inflammation, and relative rectal sparing).

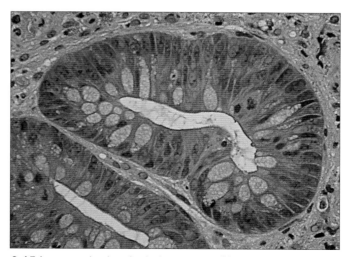

3.15 Low-grade dysplasia in a case of long-standing UC.

It should be noted that involvement of the resection margins in cases of CD does not predict a higher rate of recurrence. Two of the commonest pathological complications following surgery are diversion colitis and 'pouchitis'. The diagnosis of diversion colitis is most easily made when the mucosa is uninvolved prior to surgery. Macroscopically the mucosa ranges from almost normal to markedly inflamed. Microscopically there is characteristic striking lymphoid hyperplasia. There may be inflammatory changes with aphthous ulceration and crypt abscess formation. Even in late disease there is no architectural distortion although there may be thickening of the muscularis mucosa and externa as well as fatty and fibrous infiltration of submucosa.

Pouchitis (3.16)

There are a number of causes of inflammation in the ileal reservoir mucosa. These include infection, bacterial overgrowth, short-strip pouchitis (which may be due to exacerbation of UC in retained rectal segments of surgical anastomosis), CD (which may present as a pouch fistula or pouchitis with granulomas), and a group which shows none of the features of the above (but which is associated with colonic metaplasia). This last group may be associated with the development of dysplasia.

Microscopic features of pouchitis include:
- Ulcers with granulation tissue.
- Crypt inflammation and/or neutrophils in the lamina propria.
- Mucin depletion.
- Inconspicuous lymphoid follicles.

Pouchitis may be graded as follows:
- Type A pouch mucosa (~60%): normal small bowel histology, no/mild mucosal atrophy, no/minimal inflammation.
- Type B pouch mucosa (30–40%): transient atrophy and moderate/severe inflammation, then normalization of mucosa.
- Type C pouch mucosa (5–10%): permanent persistent atrophy and severe inflammation; well developed but still incomplete colonic-type metaplasia.

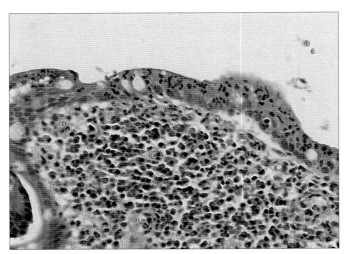

3.16 Pouchitis with active inflammation form of neutrophilic infiltrate.

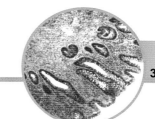

Chapter 4

Management of inflammatory bowel disease

PRINCIPLES OF MANAGEMENT AND GENERAL OBSERVATIONS

The principles of management of IBD are summarized in *Table 4.1*. Treatment is aimed at inducing clinical remission and symptomatic relief, maintaining remission, and reducing long-term complications. While there is good evidence to support some aspects of IBD therapy, the evidence in other areas is less strong and treatment may be both empirical and tailored to the individual patient.

In endeavouring to induce remission a number of factors need to be considered: extent and severity of disease, type of medication, method of administration, patient choice, and likely patient adherence to the drug regimen prescribed. These are summarized in *Table 4.2*.

Table 4.1 Principles of management of IBD

Establish the diagnosis	Exclude infection, obstruction, bile salt malabsorption, etc, or functional disease as a cause of symptoms
Induce clinical remission – Acute severe disease – Active disease	Often requires in-patient management and sometimes surgery Usually as an outpatient
Alleviate symptoms	Additional therapies such as analgesics, loperamide, etc, may be required
Maintain remission	Try to prevent relapse using 5-aminosalicylic acid or immune suppressants

Table 4.2 Factors which affect choice of therapy

Factor	Reason
Disease extent	Topical therapy may be appropriate for distal UC, or budesonide for ileal CD
Disease severity	Severe disease may require early use of oral/iv steroids Topical therapies are likely to be less effective even in distal disease if there is severe frequency of defecation
Patient adherence	Ensure the patient understands and accepts the need for medication and the proposed route of administration
Drug regimen	Immune suppressants are likely to be required in steroid-refractory or -dependent disease

Maintenance of remission

Route of administration

Clearly the route of administration is key, both in terms of efficacy and adherence. Topical therapy is effective as sole treatment for patients with restricted left-sided colonic disease, and as an adjunct to oral therapy in more extensive disease. However, if the irritation caused by administration means that using the medication is painful or the frequency of defecation means that it does not remain in the colon for any length of time, then adherence is likely to be poor. In these circumstances it is often worth considering a suppository preparation rather than a foam or liquid enema, as it is often better tolerated and is likely to remain *in situ* for longer.

Adherence

A major problem in the treatment of IBD is adherence with treatment. Studies in UC have suggested that approximately 40% of the prescribed doses of 5-aminosalicylic acid (5-ASA) treatment are actually taken by patients. Thus by improving adherence it may be possible to improve the maintenance of remission in UC. The emerging evidence that 5-ASA therapy may substantially reduce the risk of colo-rectal carcinoma in UC provides an additional reason for both patients and doctors to appreciate the importance of adherence.

Many approaches have been adopted to try and improve adherence, including more acceptable dosing regimes and patient education (*Table 4.3*). Evidence from other disease areas suggests that reducing dosing regimes from three times daily to twice daily has a major impact on adherence, and some companies have now gone on to trial once daily regimes, with good effect. There has also been a drive to identify the characteristics associated with poor adherence.

The patient's perception of the effectiveness of the medication, allied to the reasons for taking it and how they feel generally, has a significant impact on whether they take the prescribed dose. Time should be taken to explain the rationale for taking medication, especially for maintenance therapy to be taken even when the patient is well. Other strategies such as patient self-management plans and a careful exploration of any preconceptions may also help to maximize adherence to therapy.

Table 4.3 Strategies for improving patient compliance

Dosing regime	Daily or twice daily regimes are much more acceptable than thrice or more daily regimes
Acceptability of route	Rectal preparations may not be acceptable to some patients
Patient education	Careful explanation of the reasons for taking medications and the patient's perceptions
Devices	Devices to remind patients to take their medications – often electronic: probably of limited effectiveness

MANAGEMENT OF LEFT-SIDED UC

Left-sided UC is a subset of disease limited to the colon distal to the splenic flexure (**4.1**); disease limited exclusively to the rectum is referred to as ulcerative proctitis (UP).

Distal, or left-sided disease, is the commonest form of UC at presentation. Like all IBD, the course of left-sided UC varies; its onset may be gradual or abrupt with remitting and relapsing symptoms. Recognition of left-sided UC is clinically important because distal disease generally is amenable to rectally administered treatments, which work more effectively and rapidly than oral agents. Emerging data suggest that early, aggressive treatment of UC may prevent or delay proximal extension, which is commonly seen with left-sided disease (approximately 30–50% of UP will progress more proximally).

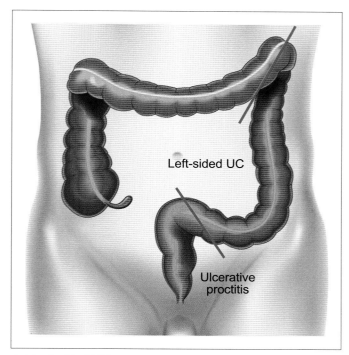

4.1 Left-sided UC.

Treatment of active left-sided UC

Rectal mesalazine preparations (5-ASAs) are the first-line treatment in view of their high efficacy and low prevalence of side-effects. Types of rectal preparations used vary depending on the extent of the disease.

Ulcerative proctitis

Mesalazine suppositories (*Pentasa*®, Salofalk®, *Asacol*®) reach the upper rectum (15–20 cm above the anal verge) and are the preferred mode of delivery for UP. Mesalazine suppositories 1 g daily for 1 month will usually control symptoms. Most patients require regular treatment to maintain remission (usually 1 g mesalazine suppository every other day or three times weekly) although a small percentage will be able to discontinue therapy without relapse.

Left-sided ulcerative colitis

Mesalazine enemas (liquid e.g. *Pentasa*® or *Salofalk*® retention enema, or foam e.g. *Asacol*® foam enema) will reach more proximally (see **4.2**). Although liquid enemas can reach the splenic flexure/distal transverse, patients often find them more difficult to administer.

Enemas are administered nightly and maximum symptomatic improvement may take 2–4 weeks. Rectally administered mesalazine preparations are effective for maintenance of remission in most patients with left-sided UC. Maintenance doses will vary from once nightly to once weekly.

In patients in whom there is significant frequency of bowel motions the enemas may not be retained, and may therefore be ineffective. Some patients may also find the

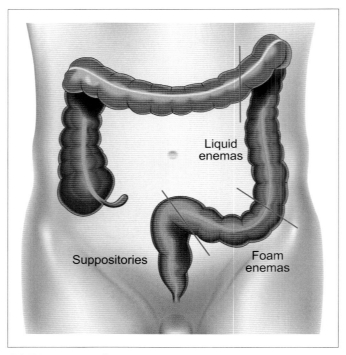

4.2 Distribution of rectally administered preparations.

foam enemas rather irritant. In these circumstances rectal preparations such as suppositories may be used if the disease is distal, liquid enemas may be substituted for foam enemas, or oral therapy may need to be instituted.

If no response occurs within 2 weeks of using a rectal mesalazine preparation, treatment with rectally administered corticosteroids (e.g. suppository *Predsol®*, or foam e.g. *Predfoam®*, or a retention enema e.g. *Predenema®*) should be added or substituted. If the steroid preparation is added one form of medication should be given in the morning and the other in the evening. Rectally administered corticosteroids on a regular basis may cause steroid-related side-effects and the benefits of prolonged therapy should be weighed against the risk in patients unresponsive to mesalazine preparations. In patients who are intolerant of mesalazine, topical corticosteroid may be used as first-line therapy.

If a combination of topical therapies proves ineffective, the addition of an oral 5-ASA to a rectal 5-ASA preparation may induce and maintain remission. This is particularly effective in patients in whom there is significant frequency of diarrhoea.

Treatment of left-sided UC refractory to 5-ASAs and rectal corticosteroids

If rectally administered 5-ASA or corticosteroids and/or oral 5-ASA therapy are not effective then oral corticosteroids are required. Prednisolone 40 mg is usually administered for 1–2 weeks and then reduced by 5 mg per week. The rate of tapering depends on disease severity and initial response, but typically would be over 8–12 weeks.

Oral and rectal 5-ASA therapy should be continued during the course of steroids and after completion, in order to maintain remission when the course of steroids is completed. It may then be possible to reduce the topical therapy, but in patients who have required oral steroid therapy, mesalazine maintenance is required, either orally or topically.

Refractory left-sided UC

There is a subgroup of patients with left-sided disease in whom symptomatic remission cannot be obtained with topical or oral mesalazine or oral prednisolone. These refractory patients pose a difficult management problem.

Patients with refractory UC should be re-evaluated to ensure correct diagnosis and disease extent, with endoscopy if necessary. There may be extension of disease more proximally or the symptoms may be caused by another condition such as a co-existing carcinoma. If the diagnosis is confirmed then it is important to consider other causes of relapses:

- Nonadherence to medication. Nonadherence to treatment regimes is a substantial problem, particularly with mesalazine, and with rectal preparations.
- 5-ASA hypersensitivity. A small proportion of patients will develop a chemical colitis caused by mesalazine or other 5-ASA compounds, and this may manifest itself as abdominal pain and diarrhoea similar to a typical UC flare.
- Infection. Superimposed infection should be excluded as a cause, by endoscopy and histology and by stool culture. *Clostridium difficile* is an increasing problem in patients with IBD, and should be excluded by early *C. difficile* testing, and endoscopy and biopsy if necessary. Other infections such as cytomegalovirus (CMV) have also been implicated in worsening underlying UC.
- Medication effects. Concurrent medications such as NSAIDs and antibiotics may trigger or exacerbate relapse of colitis.

In cases where these have been ruled out, second line therapies will be required (see below).

Steroid-dependent disease

Another group of patients may respond well to oral corticosteroid treatment, but relapse as soon as the dose is reduced, or shortly after discontinuing therapy. In this group second-line therapy similar to those with refractory disease will be required.

Second-line therapy

In patients who have confirmed active refractory ulcerative colitis or steroid-dependent disease, immune suppressants such as the thiopurines azathioprine (Aza) and 6-mercaptopurine (6-MP), or ciclosporin may be required to maintain remission in left-sided UC patients with steroid dependency. First-line therapy would normally be Aza 2–2.5 mg/kg or 6-MP 1–1.5 mg/kg after checking the thiopurine methyltransferase (TPMT) status of the patient (a key enzyme in thiopurine metabolism) to minimize the chances of developing serious side-effects, which may include leucopenia, pancreatitis, liver function abnormalities, nausea, and myalgia. The major problem with Aza is that its therapeutic effects are not normally evident for 3 months after commencing therapy. In patients who are steroid dependent, oral corticosteroids can be used to induce remission, and the dose reduced over a 3-month period. In those who have true refractory disease the mode of treatment will depend upon the severity of symptoms, and it may be necessary to consider other immune modulators such as methotrexate or ciclosporin, or anti-tumour necrosis factor (TNF) agents such as infliximab. If symptoms are severe the patient may be admitted for in-patient therapy.

Ciclosporin is not commonly used for left-sided colitis, but in exceptional circumstances may be used and can be administered as an enema, although these are difficult to use and patient compliance with treatment is poor. It may also be used intravenously and orally as a colon preserving therapy in patients who have not responded to intravenous steroid therapy for acute severe disease.

Methotrexate was originally felt to be ineffective in UC (in contrast to CD). However, more recent retrospective data have suggested it may be effective in up to 40% of UC patients refractory to other treatments. The effect may not be evident for up to 6 weeks. It may be given intra-muscularly either for the first 6 weeks or permanently, although many clinicians now give it orally once weekly, with folic acid on another day of the week to minimize the side-effects.

Infliximab offers the newest form of treatment maintenance therapy for resistant UC. Induction at 5 mg/kg (0, 2, and 6 weeks) followed by maintenance every 8 weeks will initiate response in two-thirds of patients, but the treatment is expensive, and long-term safety data are still not available.

Patients with left-sided UC or UP refractory to first- and second-line treatment, or who have acute severe colitis with systemic upset should be admitted for intravenous corticosteroid therapy (hydrocortisone 400 mg qds). Failure to respond to this or other colon-preserving therapy (ciclosporin or infliximab) may result in a proctocolectomy with end ileostomy or restorative ileal pouch anal anastomosis. Surgery is also an option for patients in whom the disease, while not medically severe, is causing an unacceptable decrease in the patient's quality of life. However, this should be discussed carefully with the patient before proceeding. For further details of medications used in UC see Part 3, Therapeutic Modalities in Inflammatory Bowel Disease.

Recommended reading

James SL, Irving PM, Gearry RB, Gibson PR. Management of distal ulcerative colitis: frequently asked questions analysis. *Intern Med J* 2008 Feb;**38**(2):114–19.

Regueiro M, Loftus EV Jr, Steinhart AH, Cohen RD. Medical management of left-sided ulcerative colitis and ulcerative proctitis: critical evaluation of therapeutic trials. *Inflamm Bowel Dis* 2006 Oct;**12**(10):979–94.

MANAGEMENT OF EXTENSIVE UC

Initial management

Extensive UC (or pancolitis) is defined as UC affecting the colonic mucosa up to and beyond the splenic flexure. In general, the therapeutic approach is determined by the severity of the symptoms. Patients with mild–moderate disease should be started on a 5-ASA compound. However, patients with moderate–severe disease should be considered for oral prednisolone therapy. An initial treatment algorithm is given in Figure **4.3** and the hierarchy of medical treatments for the treatment of extensive disease in *Table 4.4*.

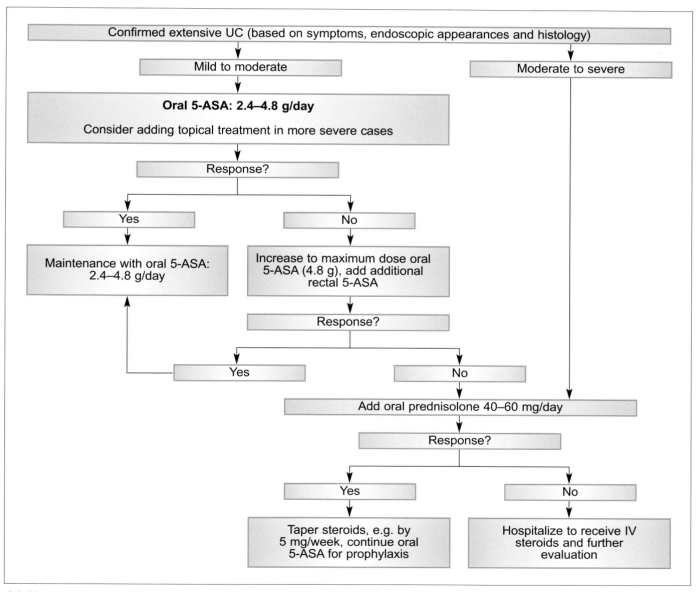

4.3 Algorithm for the initial management of extensive UC.

Table 4.4 Medications used for extensive UC

Medication	Indication	Notes
Oral 5-ASA 2.4–4.8 g daily	Mild–moderate disease	Acts on the colonic mucosa to suppress the production of pro-inflammatory mediators Dosing starts at 2.4 g increasing to 4.8 g for acute flares
Topical 5-ASA	Mild–moderate disease	Is often effective when oral therapy alone does not control symptoms This effect is seen even in extensive colitis, where the topical therapy cannot reach all of the diseased mucosa, and should be considered in patients wishing to avoid steroid therapy
Oral prednisolone 40–60 mg	Moderate–severe disease Bowel frequency >6/day with blood, and systemic upset	Full-dose therapy is continued until symptoms are completely controlled (usually 7–14 days); the dosage is then tapered gradually by 5 mg per week
Intravenous hydrocortisone	Severe disease or disease not responding to oral therapy	Dose: 100 mg qds Often given in combination with rectal therapy If no response in 3–4 days consider ciclosporin/infliximab
Aza/6-MP	Steroid-dependent disease or maintenance after treatment for severe disease	Dose: 2–3 mg/kg Aza Normally takes 3 months to see an effect Side-effects of leucopenia, pancreatitis, abnormal liver function, myalgia, and lethargy Regular blood monitoring required TPMT testing recommended before commencement
Methotrexate	Steroid-dependent disease where Aza is ineffective or not tolerated	May be started parenterally for 6 weeks and then converted to oral Normal dose 15–25 mg weekly with folic acid 5 mg daily for 3–5 days/week
Infliximab	Steroid-dependent or resistant disease where an immune suppressant is ineffective or not tolerated	Induction dose: 5 mg/kg at 0, 2, and 6 weeks and then 8 weekly maintenance Consider monotherapy rather than combination with Aza in young patients

The exact nature of the treatment options chosen needs, as always in UC, to be tailored to the patient in terms of symptoms and types of therapy used. There are a number of important points in relation to the use of different drugs in extensive UC.

Duration to wait for response

This will depend on the severity of the initial disease. If the disease is mild to moderate a greater time may be allowed for a response. However, if there is no improvement or worsening symptoms after 2 weeks further therapy should be considered. In severe disease where oral prednisolone is being used, an improvement should be sought after 1 week.

Aminosalicylates (5-ASA)

Mesalazine or another aminosalicylate is the first choice for patients with mild to moderate disease, in whom there is time to wait for a response. Other 5-ASA containing compounds include sulfasalazine and balsalazide, but mesalazine preparations are the most commonly used. The effectiveness of mesalazine as a therapy is related to the colonic mucosal concentration of the drug. This is one of the reasons that high-dose mesalazine has become more popular as a treatment for moderate UC. Doses of up to 4.8 g daily have been demonstrated to be effective in this condition, without any increase in the side-effect profile. The exact formulation of 5-ASA is less important than the dose, and it has become evident that twice daily, and possibly once daily dosing are as effective as thrice daily dosing. There is a ceiling to the amount by which mucosal concentration can be increased by oral dosing alone, and a further way to enhance mucosal concentration is the concurrent administration of both oral and rectal preparations. There is strong evidence to suggest that this combined approach is substantially more effective than oral therapy alone, even in extensive disease, where the topical therapy would not reach all the diseased mucosa. This may be because of increased mucosal concentration, and also because the extra drug in the rectum may have a disproportionate effect on urgency, one of the most distressing symptoms of UC. More physicians are prescribing combined therapy as first-line therapy in patients in whom the next therapeutic manoeuvre is likely to involve oral prednisolone to allow the maximum chance of remission with the first course of treatment.

Oral prednisolone

This should be used in patients with severe disease or moderate disease who have not responded to mesalazine, or who have systemic upset. Normal dose would be 40 mg daily, reducing once remission has been achieved, although some clinicians may use up to 60 mg daily as a starting dose. There is no evidence for the most effective way to reduce the dose, and in some patients a slow reduction (5 mg fortnightly) or a pause in the reduction regime (typically at 20 mg daily) may be appropriate. Prednisolone is ineffective as a maintenance therapy, and in patients who are steroid-dependent or who relapse quickly after tapering the dose an immune suppressant such as Aza should be considered.

Azathioprine

Aza should be considered in patients who are steroid-dependent or resistant. The drug takes 3 months to take effect, and an increasing effect may be seen up to 6 months. Thus in patients who have active disease it may be necessary to start Aza at the same time as oral prednisolone. There is much debate about whether TPMT levels should be measured before starting the drug; measurement is being done with increasing regularity and will identify patients with very low levels, who are at high risk of side-effects. It will also identify those patients in whom the level is exceptionally high, and in whom it may be appropriate to increase the dose beyond the normal range of 2–2.5 mg/kg. It is important to remember that although TPMT levels predict those at particular risk of side-effects, the majority of patients who develop side-effects on Aza have normal TPMT levels, and so regular blood monitoring remains obligatory.

Methotrexate

Methotrexate can be used as an alternative to Aza in patients who are intolerant of or resistant to Aza. Initially the evidence was thought to suggest that it was ineffective in UC, but more recent uncontrolled trials have suggested a remission rate of about 40% in UC. It may be given parenterally weekly for 6 weeks, and then converted to the oral preparation, although some clinicians start with the oral drug initially. The dose range is normally 10–25 mg weekly, with folic acid on at least 1 day when the methotrexate is not being taken. The addition of folic acid minimizes the side-effects such as mucositis, which may be very severe (see Part 3, Therapeutic Modalities in Inflammatory Bowel Disease).

Other immune suppressants

Drugs such as ciclosporin orally or tacrolimus may rarely be used in specialist centres in patients who have not responded to standard therapy; however, there is little trial evidence currently to support their use.

Infliximab

This is licensed for use in UC patients who have not responded to first-line therapy. It is expensive, with relatively poor remission rates of approximately 30%, but may be appropriate for those who cannot tolerate or fail to respond to other immune suppressants. Three doses are given to induce remission at 0, 2, and 6 weeks, at an initial dose of 5 mg/kg. However, if no effect is seen after the first dose, surgery should be considered early.

Surgery

Surgery may be considered either for patients with acute severe disease (see Chapter 12) or for patients who have persistent active disease in whom the effect of the disease on quality of life is such that the surgical options of proctocolectomy and end ileostomy or ileo-anal pouch surgery are preferable to persevering with ineffective medical therapy.

Acute severe or persistent active disease

Patients who have acute severe disease or who have persistent active disease may require admission to hospital for treatment with intravenous corticosteroid therapy. This is described further in Chapter 5, Acute, severe colitis.

Recommended reading

Brain O, Travis SP. Therapy of ulcerative colitis: state of the art. *Curr Opin Gastroenterol* 2008 Jul;24(4):469–74.

Marteau P, Probert CS, Lindgren S, *et al.* Combined oral and enema treatment with Pentasa (mesalazine) is superior to oral therapy alone in patients with extensive mild/moderate active ulcerative colitis: a randomized, double blind, placebo controlled study. *Gut* 2005 Jul;54(7):960–5.

Table 4.5 Factors affecting treatment of CD

Factor	Consequence
Discontinuous disease (skip lesions)	More than one mode of administration may be required
Rectal sparing in colonic CD	Topical therapies may be less effective than in UC
Stricturing disease	Symptoms may be due to obstruction or small bowel overgrowth rather than active inflammation
Poor response to 5-ASA therapy	5-ASA is ineffective in maintaining medically induced remission, therefore early use of Aza may be required

MANAGEMENT OF CD

Introduction

The management of CD has many similarities to that of UC, but also some significant differences. The most fundamental is that because the disease recurs after surgery there is no operative cure for CD, and surgical intervention is therefore limited to the minimum required. In addition the complications of fistulation and stricturing are much more common in CD than in UC, and so treatment has to take this into account. The major factors which affect the way Crohn's management may differ from UC are listed in *Table 4.5*.

Until recently there has been little evidence that treatment of active disease can prevent complications developing. However, recent studies, particularly those of biological therapy (anti-TNF antibody treatments) have demonstrated that over a follow-up of nearly 2 years there is a decrease in the requirement for major surgery from 38% to 14% in patients who achieve mucosal healing. This has meant that mucosal healing (as judged endoscopically), as well as symptomatic improvement, has become an important end point in the treatment of CD. This has led to a more aggressive approach to treatment, and steroid use is minimized because, although it delivers symptomatic improvement, there is no evidence that corticosteroid therapy induces significant mucosal healing. Despite this trend for more aggressive therapy it must always be remembered that some patients have relatively few complications from CD, and the possible side-effects of potent immune suppression have to be weighed up in each case so that treatment is tailored to the individual patient.

Other factors which affect the medical treatment of CD are the site or sites of disease – the presence of skip lesions may mean that there are areas of inflammation separated by normal bowel, and the medication needs to reach all sites.

Treatment of active disease

First-line therapy

The first-line treatment of active disease depends on the site of disease:

Colonic disease

The treatments are similar to those for UC. For left-sided disease topical therapy with suppositories or enemas may be used, whereas for more extensive disease systemic therapies are usually required. 5-ASA may be used first line in patients with mild symptoms, but the evidence base is not strong and for patients with mild–moderate or more severe symptoms then steroid preparations should be considered.

Ileocolonic disease

For isolated ileocolonic disease affecting only the right colon (ileocaecal disease) then 5-ASA may be considered, but as above the evidence base is small, and more effective first-line therapy would be with a 'topical' steroid such as budesonide. This is taken orally, but is formulated to release the drug in the distal small intestine. It acts locally and then 90% of the drug is metabolized by the liver, meaning that the systemic steroid effects are minimized. The normal starting dose is 9 mg daily for 4 weeks, reducing the dose subsequently. It is important to note that although there are significantly fewer steroid-related side-effects with budesonide these may still occur, and the dose should be reduced gradually in order to minimize the effects of any pituitary axis suppression. If budesonide is not effective then changing to a conventional oral corticosteroid such as prednisolone may often produce good results. An algorithm for the management of ileocaecal disease is shown in Figure **4.4**. For more extensive colonic involvement budesonide is unlikely to be effective and conventional corticosteroids can be considered first line.

Diffuse small bowel or widespread disease

First-line therapy in these circumstances will normally require systemic steroid therapy with prednisolone. This may be in conjunction with topical therapies depending on the exact areas of the gut that are affected. For patients with upper GI involvement, steroids with proton pump inhibitor therapy may be effective. Patients with extensive small bowel disease should have immune modulators introduced early in the course of disease to try to minimize longer-term problems.

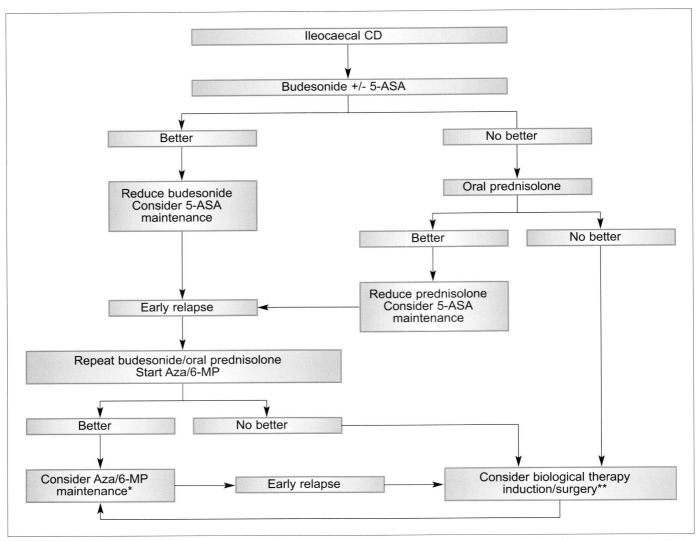

4.4 Treatment algorithm for the initial management of ileocaecal CD. In severe cases oral or iv steroids may be used initially to treat the disease. In any case the treatment should be tailored to the needs of the individual patient. With more extensive colonic involvement other treatments including topical therapies should be considered.

*Aza maintenance should be instituted in patients who have steroid-refractory or -dependent disease, and in patients post-surgery if there is endoscopic evidence of recurrence 6 months post-surgery. If induction has been induced with infliximab in Aza naïve patients then Aza maintenance should be commenced. Otherwise maintenance should be with the biological therapy.

**Surgery is an effective treatment for a short segment of ileocaecal CD, and should be considered. Biological therapy can be used in patients who have failed with immune suppressants or as a bridge to allow immune suppressants such as Aza to be commenced.

Treatment of relapsing or refractory disease

In patients with disease that relapses quickly or fails to respond to therapy (refractory disease), or those who have steroid-dependent disease the approach is very similar to that taken with UC:

- Re-evaluate the disease, with endoscopy if necessary to ensure proper diagnosis and disease extent.
- Consider other causes of relapses:
- noncompliance (especially for rectal preparations);
- 5-ASA hypersensitivity (causing a chemical colitis, manifesting as abdominal pain and diarrhoea similar to a typical UC flare);
- infection (*Clostridium difficile* should be excluded);
- medication effects (e.g. NSAIDs, antibiotics);
- misdiagnosis.

Once satisfied that the problem relates to active CD there are a number of treatment options:

- Re-treat with corticosteroids if this was effective previously, and there has been a long interval between relapses, or the relapses are mild–moderate only.
- Re-treat with corticosteroids and add an immune modulator such as Aza (or 6-MP) or methotrexate – preferred for patients who relapse quickly or who have severe or extensive disease.
- Use a biological therapy such as infliximab or adalimumab to induce remission, and maintain remission with a biological agent or an immune modulator or a combination of the two.
- Surgery – a good option for limited ileocolonic disease (ileocaecal resection), and sometimes for colonic disease behaving like UC.

Re-treating with oral corticosteroids is a possibility, but should probably be limited to those who have relapsed infrequently. For patients with frequently relapsing or steroid-dependent disease, early addition of an immune modulator such as Aza, 6-MP, or methotrexate would be recommended to induce and maintain remission.

Aza (or 6-MP) would be the standard first choice at a dose of 2–2.5 mg/kg for Aza (or 0.5–1 mg/kg for 6-MP) after checking the TPMT status of the patient to minimize the chances of developing serious side-effects, which may include leucopenia, pancreatitis, liver function abnormalities, nausea, and myalgia. The major drawback of Aza is the time to onset of clinical action, which is normally about 3 months. This means that in patients with very severe disease it is not an option to gain quick disease control. In this case either systemic steroids need to be given concomitantly, or a different agent can be used.

Methotrexate may work faster, but can still take up to 6 weeks to give a clinical effect. The best evidence is for once weekly intramuscular injection; however, some patients find this inconvenient and accordingly an oral preparation is also sometimes favoured. This is also give once weekly at a dose of 10–25 mg. Side-effects can be minimized by giving folic acid 10 mg daily for 4 days of the week, not including the day of the methotrexate dose. It cannot be used in patients who may become pregnant because of its teratogenic effects, and this means that it is not suitable for a large number of young female patients. Ciclosporin is not routinely recommended for the treatment of CD.

The use of biological therapy to induce remission should be considered in those who have failed on an immune modulator, or who are not acutely responding to steroid therapy. Some authors advocate the use of 'biologics' early in the disease, even before steroid therapy (the so-called 'top down approach'). This is not routine practice; however many do now advocate the use of biologics if steroids fail in patients who are likely to have a complicated course. This can be predicted to a certain extent from the characteristics of the disease, including those shown in *Table 4.6*. The

Table 4.6 Predictors of aggressive disease course

Diagnosis at an early age (<40 y)

Colonic or perianal involvement

Upper gastrointestinal disease

Penetrating disease type

Presence of extraintestinal manifestations

presence of these features would suggest that early introduction of immune modulation or biological therapy would be appropriate. The current biologics available are antibodies directed at TNF-α and include infliximab and adalimumab. For infliximab standard induction treatment is three doses at 5 mg/kg (0, 2, and 6 weeks) as intravenous infusions followed by maintenance infusions every 8 weeks. For adalimumab induction is with 160 mg subcutaneously followed 2 weeks later by 80 mg, or 80 mg followed by 40 mg, and then maintenance with 40 mg every other week. This has the advantage over infliximab of not requiring the patient to attend the clinic for each dose.

Biological therapies will induce a response in approximately 70% of patients, and there is now good evidence that it is more effective if given as regular maintenance therapy rather than as episodic treatments for relapses of active disease. This is thought to be because regular therapy decreases the levels of immunoglobulins directed against the therapeutic antibody.

Following the 'SONIC' trial of infliximab *vs.* Aza *vs.* a combination of infliximab and Aza in patients requiring a second course of corticosteroids, the use of combination therapy has become widespread. This trial in Aza naïve patients demonstrated that combination therapy was more effective than infliximab, which was in turn more effective than Aza in inducing and maintaining remission of up to 1 year. This difference was also seen in rates of mucosal healing. However, there remain concerns about the long-term side-effects of the combination of potent immune modulators, particularly in terms of malignancy, and many clinicians use combination therapy for the first 6 months and then use biologic monotherapy, as this may reduce the risk of complications including lymphoma (see Chapter 10, Malignancy in inflammatory bowel disease). This is because there is evidence that the first 6 months is the most crucial period in decreasing the immunogenicity of the biological treatment. The decision about treatment subsequently can then be made in consultation with the patient.

In patients who initially respond to biological therapy but then develop breakthrough symptoms, the dose intervals may be shortened or the dose increased (the former if the patient improves immediately after treatment but relapses before the next dose; the latter if there is an immediate loss of effect in a patient who originally responded).

Other drugs and treatments for active CD

5-ASA

There is some evidence for the use of 5-ASA in the treatment of active CD, but it is not compelling. In patients with mild disease, high-dose oral 5-ASA may be tried for a short period. It also probably has an effect in preventing relapse after surgery (although interestingly not after medically induced remission).

Immune suppressants

Other immune suppressants including mycophenolate mofetil have been used in open label situations in patients with refractory CD with some success, but should probably be used within specialist centres only.

Biological therapies

A number of other new biological therapies have been trialled in CD with some success including certolizumab (a fusion protein of the soluble TNF receptor) and natalizumab (anti-α4β7 integrin). Currently these are not licensed in the UK and Europe, but are likely to be in the future, and there are many other targeted biological therapies in development.

Diet

Diet has been used with great success as a treatment for CD, particularly in the paediatric population. Elemental or polymeric diets are effective (although polymeric diets are more palatable), and in paediatric patients with small bowel disease are as effective as oral steroids in inducing remission, without the significant issues that arise with steroids regarding growth retardation. They may also be effective in adults, although compliance is often poor in adults and they may relapse quickly in stopping the diet.

Antibiotics

A number of antibiotics have been used in CD, and metronidazole and ornidazole in particular have been demonstrated to be more effective than placebo. However, metronidazole is associated with a peripheral neuropathy, which may limit its long-term use, and it is advisable not to drink alcohol while taking the antibiotic. The therapeutic effect is, however, modest, and other therapies are often required in addition to these antibiotics. Other antibiotics are frequently used in the treatment of fistulizing CD, particularly with perianal fistulae. Commonly prescribed antibiotics include amoxycillin, co-amoxiclav, and ciprofloxacin.

Maintaining remission in CD

As detailed above, patients who relapse frequently should receive maintenance therapy to minimize steroid use; Aza at a dose of 2–2.5 mg/kg (or 0.5–1 mg/kg 6-MP), after checking their TPMT level, is the usual choice. If this fails to maintain adequate control then a switch to an alternative immune modulator such as methotrexate is a possibility, although many clinicians would now change to a biologic to induce and maintain remission in these patients. There is little evidence for the use of 5-ASA in CD in patients who have not undergone surgery, but it may have a role in patients with mild colonic disease. In patients who require biological therapy in order to achieve medical remission then maintenance therapy with that treatment is usually required.

Prevention of post-operative recurrence

In patients who have their macroscopic disease resected the chances of relapse are high, and treatment may be required to try to minimize this. The single most important factor is to tell patients to stop smoking, and if necessary to provide support in this endeavour. From a pharmacological viewpoint the use of 5-ASA probably has some effect and should be started in all patients after their first surgery if there is no contraindication. There is good evidence for the use of imidazole antibiotics (metronidazole or ornidazole) for 3 months after surgery in reducing post-operative recurrence; however this approach is rarely used in the UK due to the difficulty of obtaining ornidazole, and the side-effects and poor tolerability of metronidazole. After a second operation all patients should be considered for Aza maintenance therapy. Indeed after a first surgery many physicians are now assessing the disease 6–12 months after the operation, and if there are endoscopic (with aphthous ulceration) or other signs of recurrence at that stage then Aza or 6-MP maintenance therapy is commenced even in this group. There are trials ongoing to assess the effectiveness of biological therapy in this situation, but in patients who have undergone multiple resections infliximab or adalimumab maintenance therapy may be appropriate.

New therapeutic approaches

As mentioned above, the goals of therapy in CD are to try to prevent the long-term complications by aggressive early treatment in appropriate patients. It has been argued that 'top down' therapy should be the goal, particularly in high-risk groups. Advocates of this approach suggest that early treatment with biological therapy and immune modulators decreases the requirement for steroid therapy and long-term complications. Stratifying for risk of severe disease using criteria such as those in Table 4.6, may help identify patients for early use of biological therapy. The long-term results of this approach are not yet available but are eagerly awaited, and are likely to be positive given the proven benefits of biologics on mucosal healing. The important long-term issue remains the level of serious side-effects that prolonged therapy may induce.

Stopping treatment in CD

Both patients and doctors are keen to reduce medication if at all possible when the patient is well; however, it is important that this is done in a controlled way, bearing in mind the risks of relapse. All courses of steroid therapy should be time limited, and reducing in dose, so that the patient would normally aim to stop the drug within a few months. For all other therapies the decisions can be more complex.

For Aza and other immune modulators there is evidence of benefit for up to 3 years, and a trial of Aza withdrawal suggests that approximately 50% will relapse within 2 years if the drug is discontinued. However, this also means that about 50% remain in remission, thus for patients who have been well for a period of 2 or 3 years on Aza a trial of withdrawal is reasonable.

For biological therapy it is even less clear what the correct approach should be. The evidence from one trial of withdrawal of infliximab in patients in stable steroid-free remission suggests that the majority of patients relapse quickly. However, there is a group of patients with specific characteristics that relapses at a lower rate. These characteristics are shown in Table 4.7 (overleaf). In these patients it seems reasonable to try stopping the treatment. Further trials are required to lessen the uncertainty in this area.

Table 4.7 Characteristics associated with a low rate of relapse in the STORI trial on stopping infliximab

CD endoscopic index of severity (CDEIS) <2 (i.e. complete mucosal healing)

Ultrasensitive CRP <5 mg/dl

Haemoglobin >14.5 g/dl

Infliximab trough level <2 g/ml

Recommended reading

Dignass A, Van Asche G, Lindsay JO *et al.* The second European evidence-based consensus on the diagnosis and management of Crohn's disease: Current management. *J Crohn's Colitis* 2010;4;28–62.

PART 2

COMPLICATIONS AND COMORBIDITIES

Chapter 5
Acute, severe colitis

Introduction

Acute, severe colitis is characterized by bloody diarrhoea that is frequently associated with abdominal pain and systemic features such as fever and tachycardia. The lifetime risk of acute, severe colitis is about 15% in patients with UC. It tends to occur in patients with established disease, but 10% of patients present for the first time with acute, severe disease. It may also occur in patients with colonic CD. Historically, acute, severe colitis was associated with high mortality, exceeding 30%. However, in the modern era, mortality in specialist units is less than 2%. This in part reflects the implementation of intensive medical treatment such as high-dose corticosteroids, but also the earlier and better selection of patients requiring urgent colectomy. Surgical techniques and post-operative care have also undoubtedly improved.

The mainstay of treatment remains high-dose corticosteroids, but second-line or 'rescue' medical therapies are now available to try and avert the need for colectomy. One of the key clinical dilemmas posed to doctors caring for patients with acute, severe colitis is how far to persevere with intensive medical therapies, when to institute 'rescue' medical therapies, and when to elect for surgery. The possibility of preserving the colon has obvious merit. Surgery, its attendant complications and the prospect of a stoma, even temporarily, are often feared most by patients with IBD. However, procrastination in the face of

failing medical therapy and a clinically deteriorating patient leads to increased surgical complications and increased mortality. The timing of surgery has been helped by identifying a number of important clinical variables that predict which patients will probably require colectomy following an inadequate response to medical therapy. Surgery can be both curative and lifesaving. Although resistance to medical therapy is the most common reason for requiring colectomy, other specific indications in acute, severe colitis include toxic megacolon, colonic perforation, and uncontrollable haemorrhage.

Diagnosis

The diagnosis of acute, severe colitis is based on clinical and laboratory parameters. In Oxford during the 1950s, Truelove and Witt identified important criteria used to define acute, severe colitis that retain validity today. These are listed in *Table 5.1*. Additional laboratory features that corroborate the diagnosis include an elevated C-reactive protein (CRP), reduced serum albumin (<35 g/l), and an elevated platelet count, although these are nonspecific features of inflammation. The diagnosis is also supported by endoscopic visualization of the colonic mucosa confirming inflammation. Plain abdominal radiographs may reveal colonic dilatation, wall oedema (colonic wall thickening and 'thumb printing'), mucosal islands, and proximal constipation (**5.1**).

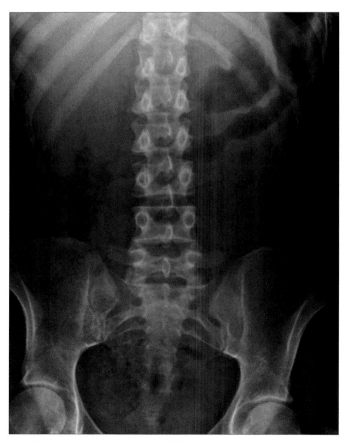

5.1 X-ray appearances of colitis – little air in the left colon with a featureless colon and wall oedema, and proximal constipation.

Table 5.1 Truelove and Witt's criteria for acute, severe colitis

Bloody diarrhoea >6 /day with one of the following:

Clinical parameter	Values in acute, severe UC
Temperature	>37.8°C
Pulse rate	>90 beats/min
Haemoglobin	<10.5 g/dl
ESR	>30 mm/hour

Additional features that may corroborate the diagnosis include elevated CRP, reduced serum albumin (<35 g/l) and an elevated platelet count

Investigations

Clinical, radiological, endoscopic, and laboratory investigations are important in the diagnosis of acute, severe colitis and also to monitor for complications and to assess response to treatment. These are summarized in *Table 5.2* and further detailed below.

Table 5.2 Investigations in acute, severe ulcerative colitis

Investigation	*Timing*	*Comments*
Stool cultures	On admission	For all patients – at least three to be sent for MC&S and *C. difficile* testing
Full blood count	On admission and daily until clinical improvement stable	
Urea and electrolytes	On admission and daily until clinical improvement stable	
CRP and ESR	On admission and daily until clinical improvement stable	CRP at day 3 helps predict the need for colectomy (>45 has an 85% chance of colectomy)
Liver function tests (inc. albumin)	On admission and at least alternate days until clinical improvement stable	
Cholesterol and magnesium	On admission	Low cholesterol (<3 mmol/l) and low magnesium (<0.5 mmol/l) are associated with fits in patients on iv ciclosporin
Thiopurine methyltransferase (TPMT)	On admission if patient may require azathioprine	
Plain abdominal X-ray	On admission and daily until clinical improvement stable	Monitor for colonic dilatation, mucosal islands, and thumb printing
CT scan	If suspicion of colonic perforation	May be used as an alternative to erect chest X-ray
Erect chest X-ray	If any suspicion of perforation or contemplating infliximab therapy	
Endoscopy	Shortly after admission Usually an unprepared flexible sigmoidoscopy	This helps to assess severity and to exclude *C. difficile* and CMV superinfection

Clinical parameters

A stool chart documenting the number of stools, consistency, and the presence of blood should be recorded daily by nursing staff or the patient. In addition to >6 bloody stools per day being one of the defining features of acute, severe colitis, serial monitoring of stool frequency is a useful prognostic marker of response to medical therapy. Criteria including the passage of >8 bloody stools at day 3 despite high-dose intravenous corticosteroids, predict an 85% probability of colectomy during the acute admission (*Table 5.3*). The vital signs, in particular temperature and pulse rate should be charted every 6 hours. Patients should be examined at least daily to assess abdominal tenderness and bowel sounds. Abdominal findings should be interpreted in the context of the possibility that high-dose corticosteroids may mask clinical signs of peritonism. For instance, patients deteriorating in all other objective respects (e.g. increasing tachycardia, unexplained acidosis) but with minimal or no abdominal signs should be regarded with suspicion. Capillary blood glucose is measured 6-hourly to monitor for glucose intolerance secondary to high-dose corticosteroid and/or ciclosporin therapy.

Laboratory parameters

Stool samples

At least three should be sent for bacterial culture and sensitivity and *Clostridium difficile* assay in all patients. More than 10% of colitis exacerbations are complicated, precipitated, or associated with colonic infection. The most commonly implicated organism is *C. difficile*. Detection of concomitant infection is especially important in patients likely to be started on powerful immunosuppressive agents such ciclosporin and tumour necrosis factor (TNF) antagonists.

Biochemical and haematological indices

These are very useful in diagnosis and monitoring response to therapy. Although serum CRP is frequently raised in exacerbations of CD, it is inconsistently elevated in acute, severe colitis. However, if it is elevated it provides a useful tool for evaluating the response to therapy and for determining prognosis. The Oxford group have demonstrated that 85% of patients subsequently required colectomy during the acute admission, if serum CRP concentration remained >45 mg/l following 3 days of intensive intravenous corticosteroid therapy. Serum albumin concentration is often negatively associated with acute, severe colitis and a low serum concentration also independently predicts failure of intensive medical therapy. The criteria predicting colectomy are listed in *Table 5.3*.

Table 5.3 Travis criteria for severe UC

Assessment at day 3

If bowel frequency is >8/day
OR
Bowel frequency 3–8/day with a CRP of >45 mg/l

Risk of colectomy is >85%

These patients should have early second-line therapy for acute, severe UC

Close monitoring of serum electrolytes is necessary, with particular emphasis on potassium, which is prone to depletion from excess faecal losses. Serum magnesium and cholesterol concentrations should be measured in anticipation of potential ciclosporin therapy. Intravenous ciclosporin is associated with epileptiform seizures and the risk is greatest in patients with hypomagnesaemia (<0.5 mmol/l) and hypocholesterolaemia (<3.0 mmol/l).

In patients who have not previously been treated with azathioprine (Aza) it is sensible to send a thiopurine methyltransferase level (TPMT) on admission, as this predicts patients who may develop side-effects from Aza, and most patients who respond to medical therapy for acute, severe colitis will be discharged on Aza.

Haemoglobin concentration is frequently reduced in acute, severe colitis secondary to blood loss and chronic disease. An elevated platelet count and erythrocyte sedimentation rate (ESR) are nonspecific markers of inflammation. Changes in ESR frequently lag behind clinical response and consequently are considered less reliable markers of disease activity and response to treatment compared to CRP, which has a half-life of only 19 hours and also becomes elevated earlier.

Radiological and endoscopic parameters

Daily plain abdominal X-rays are recommended to assess the development of complications such as toxic dilatation. Colonic dilatation is defined as a maximal colonic diameter of >5.5 cm in the transverse colon, or >9 cm in the caecum, which has a thinner wall and dilates more readily (**5.2**). Colonic dilatation persisting for >24 hours indicates a high likelihood of imminent perforation and is an indication for urgent colectomy. In addition to diagnosing the extent of disease and identifying complications such as toxic megacolon, plain abdominal radiology is also useful for determining prognosis. Small bowel dilatation (indicating ileus), colonic dilatation, and identification of mucosal islands all predict failure of medical therapy and likelihood of requiring colectomy. An erect chest radiograph and/or abdominal computed tomography (CT) scan are the investigations of choice if colonic perforation is suspected. A baseline chest X-ray is also obligatory when contemplating anti-TNF therapy, to evaluate possible exposure to tuberculosis. With the advent of widespread access to endoscopy, air contrast barium enema is seldom employed to diagnose and assess acute, severe colitis.

5.2 Wall oedema and colonic dilatation on an X-ray of a patient with acute severe UC.

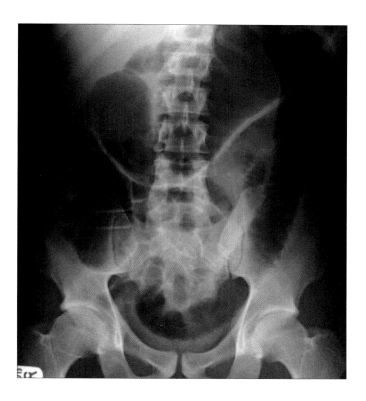

There are theoretical safety concerns regarding endoscopy in the setting of acute, severe colitis. There is a perceived risk of colonic perforation in friable, inflamed colonic tissue secondary to high volume air insufflation and endoscope trauma. Most gastroenterologists favour unprepared flexible sigmoidoscopy rather than colonoscopy in patients with severe inflammation in an attempt to minimize these theoretical risks. Endoscopy allows direct visualization of colonic mucosa and allows objective assessment of colonic inflammation (5.3). Endoscopy also provides the opportunity to acquire mucosal biopsies for histological assessment. This is particularly useful in patients presenting for the first time with acute, severe disease in order to differentiate between UC, CD, and other causes of colonic inflammation such as infection, ischaemia, and vasculitis. Biopsies are important to exclude superimposed infections such as cytomegalovirus (CMV) or *C. difficile*. It is important to remember that up to 15% of *C. difficile* cases may be toxin negative, and so histology may be important in confirming the diagnosis.

Treatment

Patients with acute, severe colitis should be admitted to hospital for intensive treatment and close monitoring. Combined responsibility from medical and surgical teams is necessary to assess clinical progress, response to medical therapy, development of complications, timing and appropriateness of second-line medical therapies and, if necessary, the need for surgical intervention. An algorithm for the treatment of acute, severe colitis is shown in Figure **5.4**. After diagnosis patients should be commenced on *high-dose corticosteroid therapy*. Most units favour an intravenous regime, such as hydrocortisone 100 mg qds. Other intravenous corticosteroid regimes include methylprednisolone and betamethasone. Some clinicians advocate topical corticosteroid therapy administered as enemas or constant rectal instillation, in addition to systemic therapy. Intensive corticosteroids induce remission in about 60% of patients within 5–7 days. Following induction of remission, patients can be commenced on oral

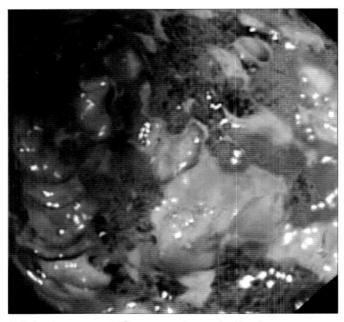

5.3 Acute, severe UC seen endoscopically; deep ulceration with islands of remaining mucosa.

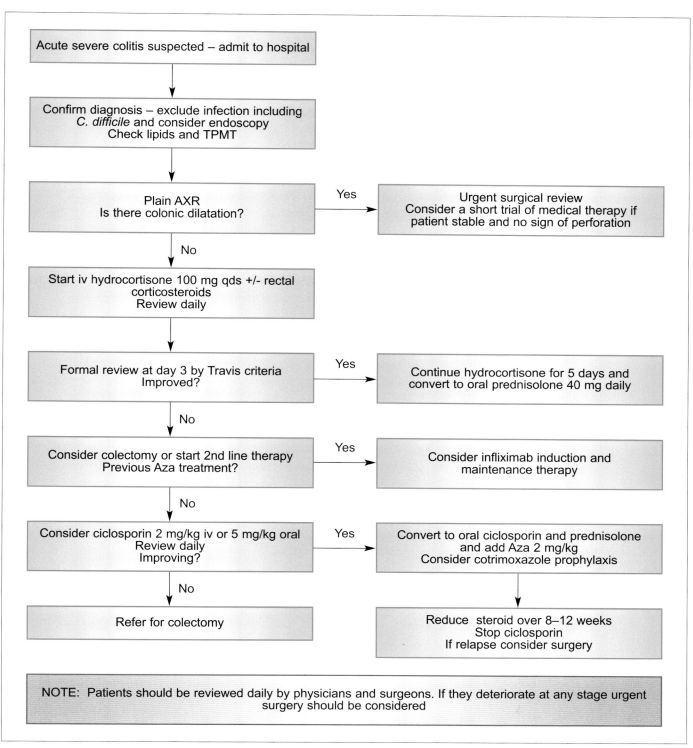

5.4 Algorithm for the management of acute, severe UC.

corticosteroids that are sequentially reduced over 3 months, often with concomitant addition of Aza therapy. Patients with no or inadequate response to systemic corticosteroids require either rescue therapy or colectomy.

In addition to intensive intravenous corticosteroid therapy, a number of nonspecific measures are also implemented. Physiological optimization is desirable, particularly in view of the relatively high likelihood of requiring surgical intervention and the attendant possibility of general anaesthesia. Measures include rehydration, potassium supplementation (aiming to keep serum concentration >4 mmol/l), and blood transfusion (aiming to keep blood haemoglobin concentration >10 g/dl). Subcutaneous low molecular weight heparin or intravenous unfractionated heparin should be prescribed as adjunctive therapy, unless severe colonic haemorrhage is present. Heparins possess anti-inflammatory activity *in vitro*, in addition to their antithrombotic properties. There are numerous open label studies, small case series, and some randomized trials, mostly evaluating the effects of heparin in less severe forms of colitis. There are no robust, randomized, placebo-controlled trials published evaluating the role of heparin in combination with standard high-dose, intensive corticosteroid therapy in acute, severe colitis. However, hospitalized medical patients with hyper-coagulable states, such as acute, severe colitis, should probably be treated with heparin as prophylaxis against venous thromboembolism. In addition to deep vein thrombosis and pulmonary embolism, acute, severe colitis has also been associated with rare thrombotic complications such as cerebral venous thrombosis. Oral low molecular weight heparins formulated as colonic release preparations are currently being evaluated in clinical trials in active colitis.

Nutritional support

Patients with acute, severe colitis may continue to eat and drink. Evidence from controlled trials of patients receiving intensive corticosteroid therapy for acute, severe colitis suggests that there is no difference in outcome measures, such as colectomy or mortality rates, in patients treated with parenteral nutrition and bowel rest compared to patients receiving normal oral nutrition. Some patients prefer not to, or are unable to eat because of nausea and pain during the acute phase of illness, and some clinicians use relapse of symptoms following reintroduction of food as an indication of medical therapy failure. Nutritional supplementation, including parenteral nutrition, can be considered in patients with marked pre-existing malnutrition, or in patients unable to tolerate oral nutrition because of nausea or vomiting for prolonged periods.

Antibiotic therapy

There is no role for blind antibiotic therapy in patients with acute, severe colitis, unless it is complicated by concomitant GI infection. Various intravenous antibiotic regimes, including ciprofloxacin monotherapy, and combined metronidazole and tobramycin therapy have been assessed in randomized, placebo-controlled trials and have not demonstrated any additional efficacy on top of high-dose intravenous corticosteroids. Isolation of pathogenic organisms, or *C. difficile* in stool samples should prompt the use of antimicrobial therapy. Antibiotics should also be considered in patients presenting for the first time with fulminant disease when an infectious aetiology is difficult to exclude. This may be relevant in patients with rapidly progressive disease in whom stool cultures have yet to yield growth, and colonic histology is either unavailable or nondiagnostic.

Second-line or 'rescue' therapy

Approximately 40% of patients with acute, severe colitis do not respond adequately to intensive intravenous corticosteroid therapy. The therapeutic options to consider in these patients include urgent colectomy or second-line, 'rescue' medical therapy.

It is important that in planning medical treatment of acute, severe colitis the patient needs to be reassessed frequently, and if there is any deterioration then surgery should be considered. Second-line therapy should be considered at day 3: if the patient has failed to respond or is deteriorating then second-line treatment should be commenced immediately. There are criteria at day 3 which may help to predict those who will need colectomy, and therefore early second-line treatment (see *Table 5.3*). Most complications and morbidity result from patients languishing on failing medical treatments for long periods, and so decisions about second-line treatment and surgery need to be taken in a timely manner.

Ciclosporin

The first widely available rescue medical therapy was intravenous ciclosporin. Ciclosporin is a fungus derived polypeptide immunosuppressant. It is a powerful inhibitor of T lymphocyte proliferation and cytokine production. The first randomized, placebo controlled trial assessing the efficacy of ciclosporin in patients with acute, severe colitis with an inadequate response to corticosteroids was reported in the early 1990s from two centres in the United States. Although this study was only conducted on 20 patients (11 receiving active drug and 9 receiving placebo) it is the most commonly cited evidence base for this treatment modality. In this study clinical response occurred in 82% (9/11) of patients receiving ciclosporin, compared to 0% (0/9) in the placebo arm. Clinical response to ciclosporin also occurred rapidly (mean 7 days). This trial was terminated early, because it was considered unethical to withhold the active drug given its apparent superior efficacy. Subsequently, patients initially randomized to receive placebo were also offered open label ciclosporin, so long-term data regarding the efficacy of ciclosporin at preventing colectomy in the long–medium term were uninterpretable. Numerous case series and retrospective analyses of intravenous ciclosporin rescue therapy have since been published, and in general it is felt that about 60% of patients may avoid colectomy in the short term, although up to 50% of the initial responders may

Table 5.4 Side-effects of ciclosporin therapy

Side-effect	Patients affected (%)
Paraesthesia	51
Hypertension	43
Nephrotoxicity	23
Infection	20
Seizures	3
Death	2

require colectomy in the following year, and its long-term efficacy remains controversial.

Critics contend that colectomy is only deferred rather than averted in many patients, and even when ciclosporin is effective it may be associated with unacceptable side-effects. In one study of 111 patients, side-effects recorded in patients receiving intravenous ciclosporin included those listed in *Table 5.4*. Strategies to reduce side-effects include using 2 mg/kg per 24 hours rather than 4 mg/kg. This appears to be equally effective, with a much better side-effect profile, and is the current recommended dose. However, levels should be checked and patients with low (<100 ng/ml) levels should have the dose increased. Identification and correction of patients with hypomagnesaemia and exclusion of patients with hypocholesterolaemia also reduce the likelihood of seizure in patients treated with intravenous ciclosporin.

Another contentious issue surrounding rescue ciclosporin therapy concerns whether to stop or continue intensive corticosteroid therapy once ciclosporin has been commenced. In the early trials, corticosteroids were continued for the duration of the ciclosporin infusion. However, there is conflicting evidence as to whether there is additional benefit from continuing corticosteroid therapy. There is also now evidence from small trials that ciclosporin monotherapy may be an effective first-line alternative to corticosteroid therapy; however, this is not currently standard practice.

Practically, ciclosporin (2 mg/kg/day) is infused either continuously, or over 6 hours, until the patient responds clinically and can take medication orally. Oral therapy (5–8 mg/kg/day in 2 divided doses) is then commenced for 3–6 months. A microemulsion preparation called Neoral® is available with better and more predictable gastrointestinal absorption. Azathioprine (2–2.5 mg/kg) or 6-mercaptopurine (6-MP) (1–1.5 mg/kg) should also be prescribed prior to discharging the patient from hospital to increase the likelihood of long-term remission. This strategy has been termed 'bridging' therapy because thiopurines may take up to 3 months before their therapeutic activity is clinically relevant. Evidence from small studies suggests that the addition of Aza to ciclosporin before discharge may significantly improve outcomes, with 80% colectomy-free at 1 year and 60% at 7 years in one Italian study. Drug level monitoring is also required with ciclosporin: a whole blood concentration of between 100 and 200 ng/ml is desirable. This can be pushed higher in the absence of side-effects in order to gain in efficacy, but patients must be closely monitored in centres used to dealing with this drug. Following institution of therapy blood levels should initially be monitored weekly for the first 2 weeks and then monthly for the remainder of treatment. Blood pressure, renal function, liver function, and clinical assessment for the development of neuropathy, particularly paraesthesias, should be specifically sought throughout the treatment period.

Biological therapies

Biological therapies, such as specific TNF antagonists, are attracting considerable interest as second-line rescue therapies. A pivotal study performed in Scandinavia in 2005 demonstrated safety and efficacy of infliximab in acute, severe colitis. Patients not responding after 3 days of high-dose intravenous corticosteroid therapy were randomized to receive either a single intravenous infusion of infliximab (5 mg/kg) or placebo. The number of patients who came to colectomy within 3 months of the infusion was 29% in the infliximab group compared with 67% in the placebo group. There were no significant side-effects observed in the infliximab-treated group and reassuringly there was no increased risk of surgical complications in patients receiving infliximab who ultimately required colectomy. Retrospective, cohort studies and published case series from the United States, the UK and Italy have also broadly corroborated these trial data in routine clinical practice. However, infliximab therapy for acute, severe colitis is not free from controversy. A well conducted, randomized placebo-controlled trial conducted in four centres in the UK and Germany assessing the efficacy of infliximab in patients with severe UC refractory to corticosteroids, failed to show any significant benefit of infliximab compared to placebo. It has been suggested that infliximab should be the rescue therapy of choice in patients who have previously failed to respond to Aza therapy, and ciclosporin in Aza-naïve patients. This is based on the long-term options available: patients in whom ciclosporin induces remission will need additional medication, normally in the form of Aza, in order to maintain long-term remission. It is therefore probably more appropriate to treat patients who have already failed Aza with infliximab rather than ciclosporin, as this can be continued as maintenance therapy after the acute episode.

It is likely that other novel therapies will become available as rescue therapy in the near future. Biological therapies engineered to antagonize specific molecular targets believed to be important in the pathogenesis of colitis are particularly attractive options with much promise. Therapies already on the horizon include interleukin-2 receptor blocking monoclonal antibodies (basiliximab and daclizumab), anti-CD3 monoclonal antibodies (visilizumab), and antibodies that inhibit circulating leukocyte adhesion to vascular endothelium, consequently preventing migration of inflammatory cells into inflamed organs (natalizumab). Leucocyophoresis, where granulocytes or lymphocytes are preferentially extracted from extracorporeal blood, and novel immunosuppressants, such as tacrolimus, are other future possibilities.

Third-line therapy

If second-line rescue therapy fails it is nearly always appropriate to proceed to surgery. Very occasionally ciclosporin and infliximab have been used sequentially but this is fraught with danger. Because of the long half-life of infliximab it is not possible to use ciclosporin after infliximab fails, and the use of infliximab after ciclosporin is also not recommended. This is because delaying surgery too long is a key factor in increasing mortality, and the combination of potent immune suppressants is likely to result in a stormy post-operative course if surgery is required. One small study found post-operative complication rates of 80% in patients who had received both infliximab and ciclosporin.

Surgery

Resection of the colon offers a cure for UC and may be life saving. In UC the operation of choice remains colectomy even in the presence of isolated left-sided disease. The results of segmental colectomy, where only the diseased portion is resected, are largely very disappointing, with rapid and often severe recurrence in the previously unaffected segment. This may lead to significant complications and the need for total colectomy fraught with the complications attendant upon operating in patients with severe disease.

Indications for surgery include toxic megacolon, perforation, uncontrolled haemorrhage, and lack of response to medical therapy. In practice, the timing of colectomy is often a more complex clinical dilemma. In some patients the response to medical therapy is slow or only partial. In these patients the clinical choices available include persevering with intensive medical therapy, implementing 'salvage' medical therapies such as ciclosporin A or anti-TNF therapies, or offering colectomy. This clinical decision is based on the opinion and experience of the attending physician and surgeon, in the context of the wishes of the appropriately counselled and informed patient. As discussed earlier, there are objective criteria to help in this decision-making, and these are summarized in *Table 5.3*.

In most circumstances the safest and simplest surgical procedure for the patient with fulminant colitis is a simple subtotal colectomy (STC) with an end-ileostomy. This procedure can now be performed laparoscopically. Many patients are unhappy with the prospect of a long term stoma and frequently desire restoration of continence. The most commonly performed restorative procedure is termed the ileal pouch anal anastamosis (IPAA) or 'ileoanal pouch'. This procedure requires a number of operations beginning at colectomy. After a recovery period from the initial combined insult of surgery and severe colitis, the terminal ileum is fashioned into a 'pouch' by joining parallel loops of ileum before anastamosis to the anus. The anastamosed loops of ileum that are formed into a pouch have sufficient volume to serve as a reservoir for faeces, analogous to the rectum.

Although colectomy does offer a cure for UC, IPAA and other restorative pouch procedures are associated with significant complications. Patients frequently experience diarrhoea with the need to defecate 4–6 times a day. The newly formed pouch is also prone to inflammation, or 'pouchitis'. Patients with pouchitis develop symptoms analogous to proctitis, including faecal urgency, passage of mucus, rectal bleeding, and faecal incontinence. Other significant complications of IPAA include infertility in both men and women and ultimately pouch failure with the need for surgical revision.

Specialist nursing

Specialist IBD and stoma nurses, where available, should be involved in the care of hospitalized patients early and for the duration of the admission. The uncounselled patient often harbours unfavourable and unsubstantiated fears regarding surgery and stomas. Experienced specialist nurses follow patients through both 'medical' and 'surgical' phases of acute, severe disease and are often a useful bridge between the two specialities. Stoma nurses can also offer objective and honest information regarding stomas.

Recommended reading

Jakobovits SL, Travis SP. Management of acute severe colitis. *Br Med Bull* 2006 Jul 17;**75–76**:131–44.

Järnerot G, Hertervig E, Friis-Liby I, *et al.* Infliximab as rescue therapy in severe to moderately severe ulcerative colitis: a randomized, placebo-controlled study. *Gastroenterology* 2005 Jun;**128**(7):1805–11.

Travis SP, Farrant JM, Ricketts C, *et al.* Predicting outcome in severe ulcerative colitis. *Gut* 1996 Jun;**38**(6):905–10.

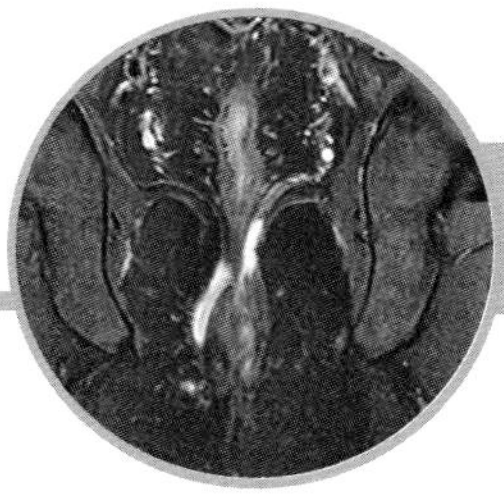

Perianal and fistulizing Crohn's disease

Perianal disease

Some of the most distressing and difficult complications of CD relate to fistulae and perianal disease. These can cause the patient pain and embarrassment, leading to social isolation and, if extensive, may cause significant malnutrition.

Disease affecting the perianal region occurs in 10–20% of CD patients. It may occur in isolation or with disease at a distant site, or in association with rectal disease. The major perianal complications are listed in *Table 6.1*. A fissure or single abscess may be treated in the conventional way by incision and drainage, but it is important to allow the abscess to drain freely.

The major forms of perianal fistulae are shown in Figure **6.1**. The management of fistulae depends upon the type of fistula and whether it is associated with local rectal inflammation. Hence the first step in the management of fistulizing disease is to delineate the extent of the disease by careful history and physical examination, endoscopic assessment of the underlying CD, and imaging of the fistulae. The most effective forms of noninvasive imaging are MRI scanning (**6.2, 6.3**) and endoscopic ultrasound (EUS). If there is any doubt, a careful examination under anaesthetic is an excellent way of delineating the extent of fistulizing disease and should be performed in most cases as an addition to noninvasive imaging. Of particular importance in the assessment is the identification of sepsis. Any collections should be drained and steps taken to maintain drainage. This may include the insertion of Seton drains through fistulous tracks to keep them open and allow pus to drain.

Table 6.1 Common perianal manifestations of CD

Perianal abscess

Perianal fissure

Isolated perianal fistula

Complex perianal fistulae

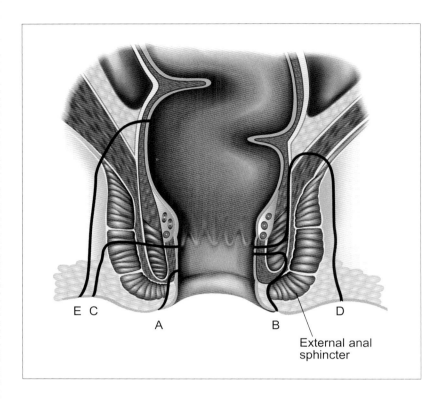

E C

A

B

D

External anal sphincter

6.1 Park's classification of perianal fistulae. A superficial fistula tracks below both the internal anal sphincter and external anal sphincter complexes (A). An inter-sphincteric fistula tracks between the internal anal sphincter and the external anal sphincter in the inter-sphincteric space (B). A trans-sphincteric fistula tracks from the inter-sphincteric space through the external anal sphincter (C). A supra-sphincteric fistula leaves the inter-sphincteric space over the top of the puborectalis and penetrates the levator muscle before tracking down to the skin (D). An extra-sphincteric fistula tracks outside of the external anal sphincter and penetrates the levator muscle into the rectum (E). (Modified with permission from: Parks AG, Gordon PH, Hardcastle JD. A classification of fistula-in-ano. *Br J Surg* 1976;**63**(1): 1–12.) (A) and (B) are simple fistulae, (C)–(E) are complex fistulae.

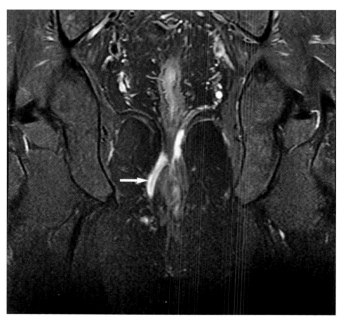

6.2, 6.3 MRI scans demonstrating complex perianal fistulae. These demonstrate branching horseshoe fistulae crossing the sphincters in sagittal (**6.2**, arrow) and coronal (**6.3**, arrow, opposite page) views.

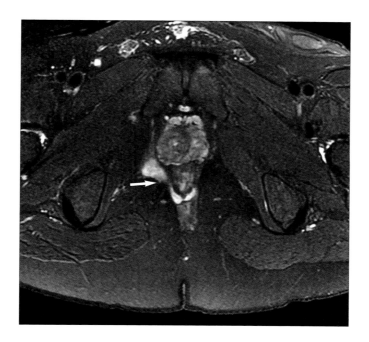

Subsequent management will depend on whether the fistulae are simple (not involving the sphincters (A and B in **6.1**)) or complex, and if they are simple whether there is any associated active rectal CD.

Simple fistulae should be treated initially with antibiotics, such as amoxicillin, co-amoxiclav, or metronidazole, and immune suppressants such as azathioprine (Aza) or 6-mercaptopurine (6-MP). These drugs will take up to 3 months to have significant therapeutic effect, and so should be started early. In patients who fail to respond then infliximab or other biological therapy such as adalimumab may be used. Trial data suggest that about 50% of patients treated with biological therapy for fistulizing disease will achieve complete closure of all fistulae after 6 months, and about 60–70% will have significant improvement in the number of draining fistulae.

In the presence of active rectal disease then the treatment of simple fistulae is similar, but biological therapy may be used early in the process to induce remission. Thus antibiotics should be started and infliximab or adalimumab used to induce remission (inflixmab 5 mg/kg at weeks 0, 2, and 6 or adalimumab 80 mg followed by 40 mg or 160 mg followed by 80 mg 2 weeks later). Immune suppressants such as Aza should be started simultaneously for maintenance therapy.

For complex fistulizing disease a combined surgical–medical approach is needed. Careful surgical evaluation with drainage of sepsis and laying open of tracts may be required, often with the placement of Seton drains. Aggressive medical therapy with biological therapy should then be used to try to aid healing, and to heal any mucosal disease, and immune suppressants should be started.

In patients who fail to respond, further medical therapy may be instituted with drugs such as tacrolimus, although the evidence base is small; in patients with very active mucosal disease associated with fistulae, surgical defunctioning of the bowel with either a defunctioning colostomy or ileostomy may be considered. In a small number of very severe cases proctectomy may be considered.

The treatment options for fistulizing perianal CD are shown in Figure **6.4**.

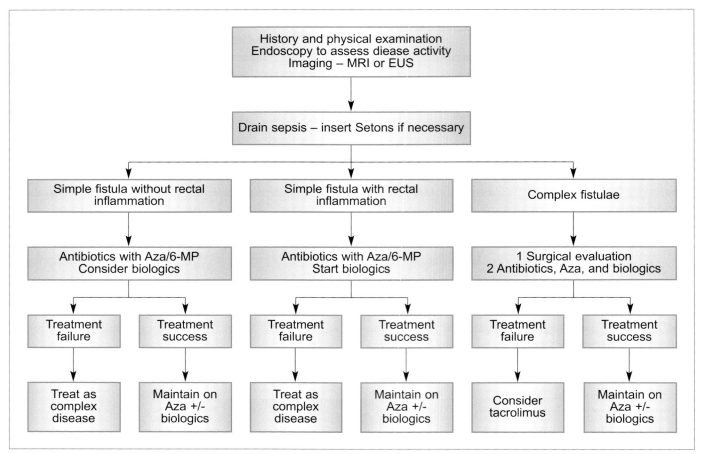

6.4 Treatment algorithm for perianal fistulae.

Fistulizing CD: special situations

Rectovaginal fistulae

Recovaginal fistulae can be extremely distressing for patients. They may present with the passage of a faeculent discharge per vagina, and the fistula may cause pain and discomfort. They are often extremely difficult to treat. Initial therapy is as for other fistulae, but they normally require surgical repair. However, there is a high level of recurrence after surgery, and concomitant treatment with biological therapy may help minimize this. In difficult cases, defunctioning of the bowel, and possibly major reconstructive surgery may be required. This often requires the input of a plastic surgeon.

Colovesical fistulae

Patients may present with pneumaturia (air bubbles in the urine) or passing gritty matter in the urine, giving rise to repeated urinary tract infections. Treatment is normally surgical to close the fistula and separate the adherent bowel from the bladder.

Entero-enteric fistulae and enterocutaneous fistulae

Entero-enteric and enterocutaneous fistulae may cause significant problems, particularly in relation to nutrition.

Entero-enteric fistulae occur when two segments of bowel apposed to each other form an abnormal connection (normally secondary to inflammation). This may allow the contents of the gut to bypass a very significant portion of the bowel length. This leads to two potential problems – firstly, because the gut contents bypass a large segment of the bowel, there is malabsorption. Secondly, the bypassed segment can become overgrown with bacteria (small bowel overgrowth), and this can exacerbate the problems of malnutrition. Thus patients may present with weight loss, steatorrhoea, low calcium or magnesium, and other signs of specific nutritional deficiencies.

Enterocutaneous fistulae may occur if surgical wounds break down or simply by erosion through the abdominal wall of severe mucosal inflammation. These patients may have similar problems with malabsorption and malnutrition, but in addition may become very dehydrated as the output from the fistulae can be very high. This may necessitate collection of the fluids in a stoma bag.

The management of these fistulae requires careful evaluation of the anatomy of the fistulae, in particular in relation to the activity of the underlying CD. This may require small bowel imaging with radiological enteroclysis or fistulograms or MRI scanning and possibly endoscopic examination through large fistulae.

The nutritional and fluid status of the patient is paramount. If there is a large volume of fluid being lost then intravenous fluids may be required if enteral fluids are insufficient. Assistance with feeding may be required depending on the site of the fistula. Ideally this should be via enteral feeding with supplemental polymeric or elemental feed, but if the fistula is very high in the proximal small bowel then parenteral nutrition may be required to maintain the patient's nutritional status.

Definitive treatment of the fistula is usually surgical. Biological therapy may be used, although the number of entero-enteric and enterocutaneous fistulae in clinical trials of fistulizing disease was small. However, use of infliximab or adalimumab may result in healing, and avoid unnecessary surgery. It may also decrease the inflammatory load prior to surgery to improve the chances of long-term success. The use of steroid treatment should be avoided if at all possible as this increases post-operative complications and negatively affects healing.

Definitive surgery should be undertaken when the patient's nutritional status has been optimized, and the anatomy of the fistula and activity of the bowel disease has been as fully assessed as possible. Maintenance therapy after surgery may be required with biological or immune suppressant therapy.

Recommended reading

Andreani SM, Dang HH, Grondona P, Khan AZ, Edwards DP. Rectovaginal fistula in Crohn's disease. *Dis Colon Rectum* 2007 Dec;**50**(12):2215–22.

Caprilli R, Gassull MA, Escher JC, *et al*; European Crohn's and Colitis Organisation. European evidence based consensus on the diagnosis and management of Crohn's disease: special situations. *Gut* 2006 Mar;**55**(Suppl 1):i36–58.

Felley C, Mottet C, Juillerat P, *et al*. Fistulizing Crohn's disease. *Digestion* 2007;**76**(2):109–12.

Schwartz DA, Herdman CR. Review article: The medical treatment of Crohn's perianal fistulas. *Aliment Pharmacol Ther* 2004 May 1;**19**(9):953–67.

Chapter 7

Microscopic colitis

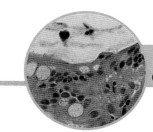

Introduction

Microscopic colitis is a term that is generally taken to refer to two conditions – collagenous colitis and lymphocytic colitis. In these conditions there is microscopic evidence of inflammation in the context of a normal colonoscopic examination. The conditions are probably not linked to UC and CD, but may cause chronic symptoms, and are thus included.

Both collagenous and lymphocytic colitis tend to present in middle age, with collagenous colitis being significantly more common in females. The clinical features are listed in *Table 7.1*, but the most significant is normally watery diarrhoea without the presence of blood. When it is active the diarrhoea typically occurs 4–8 times a day, although it can be more frequent in severe cases.

The patient may suffer from constant symptoms or the diarrhoea may be intermittent, occurring in repeating cycles. The cause of microscopic colitis is not known, but as with UC and CD it may be related to luminal microbiota, and there are reports of familial clustering suggesting that genetic influences may be important. Microscopic colitis is also associated with a number of autoimmune disorders, most notably coeliac disease. These associations are listed in *Table 7.2*.

Table 7.1 Clinical features of microscopic colitis

Chronic diarrhoea

Abdominal pain or cramps

Abdominal bloating

Modest weight loss

Nausea

Faecal incontinence

Dehydration

Table 7.2 Autoimmune disorders associated with microscopic colitis

Diabetes mellitus

Rheumatoid arthritis

Thyroid disorders

Pernicious anaemia

Scleroderma

Sjögren's syndrome

CREST syndrome

Medications have also been implicated as possible risk factors for microscopic colitis, particularly NSAIDs, but including other commonly prescribed drugs. It is therefore very important to take a thorough drug history in patients with microscopic colitis.

Diagnosis of microscopic colitis depends upon a high index of suspicion based on the clinical history, together with a colonoscopy with biopsies. The diagnosis rests upon an essentially normal colonoscopy with microscopic evidence of colitis. About 30–40% of patients will have disease proximal to the sigmoid colon, so a flexible sigmoidoscopy is not sufficient to exclude the diagnosis, and multiple biopsies should be taken as the colitis may be patchy.

Microscopically the two types of colitis are distinct: in collagenous colitis there is inflammation with lymphocytic infiltration of the colon and marked thickening of the collagen band which lies just below the colonic epithelium. This is normally present, but is thickened in collagenous colitis (**7.1**). Lymphocytic colitis is characterized by the presence of increased numbers of intraepithelial lymphocytes but without evidence of thickening of the collagen band (**7.2**).

Treatment of microscopic colitis is largely empirical as there have been few trials of therapy.

Lifestyle adjustments

Dietary adjustments may help, including restricting fat intake, a lactose-free diet, and reducing intake of caffeine and soft drinks. Patients should be advised not to use NSAIDs.

Medical therapies

Often symptomatic treatment with antidiarrhoeal agents such as loperamide are used, particularly if the symptoms are mild. Sometimes treatment with bile acid sequestrants such as cholestyramine may improve diarrhoea symptoms, although they may also cause bloating. Specific therapies include mesalazine (5-ASA) or bismuth subsalicylate (Pepto-bismol®) may be used. Treatment with mesalazine is effective in approximately 50% of cases, and there is a small open-label trial of bismuth in patients with lymphocytic colitis, suggesting a benefit in up to 60% of patients.

If these therapies fail then steroid therapy may be required. Budesonide is often used first line as it is associated with fewer systemic side-effects than prednisolone. However, in severe cases prednisolone or even immune suppressant therapy with azathioprine (Aza) or methotrexate may occasionally be required. Symptoms frequently relapse upon cessation of treatment with steroids.

The long-term prognosis for microscopic colitis is generally good. Surgery for active disease is very rarely required, and patients do not tend to encounter the long-term sequelae seen in UC and CD. In particular there appears to be no increased risk of colonic carcinoma, and strictures and fistulae do not occur. Symptoms tend to improve with time, and in a large proportion of patients may resolve completely, while in others they may pursue a relapsing and remitting course.

Recommended reading

Pardi DS. After budesonide, what next for collagenous colitis? *Gut* 2009 Jan;**58**(1):3–4.

Tangri V, Chande N. Microscopic colitis: an update. *J Clin Gastroenterol* 2009 Apr;**43**(4):293–6.

Tysk C, Bohr J, Nyhlin N, Wickbom A, Eriksson S. Diagnosis and management of microscopic colitis. *World J Gastroenterol* 2008 Dec 28;**14**(48):7280–8.

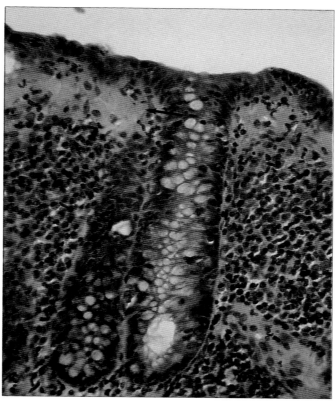

7.1 Collagenous colitis. There is a widened collagen band just beneath the epithelium showing as a band of light pink staining material (arrow).

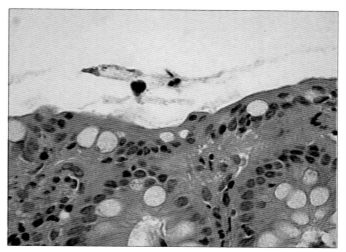

7.2 Lymphocytic colitis. The epithelium has increased numbers of lymphocytes within it.

Chapter 8

Fertility and inflammatory bowel disease

Introduction

Research has suggested that the infertility rate among females with UC and quiescent CD prior to surgery is no different to that of the general population, although females with active CD have been reported to have some impairment in fertility. Men with UC have normal fertility compared to the general population but there is some evidence that fertility is reduced in men with CD. Men undergoing restorative proctocolectomy (RPC) for UC may suffer from retrograde ejaculation and erectile dysfunction; however, male sexual function has been reported to improve following RPC.

A meta-analysis of eight studies and systematic review of 22 studies has reported that females have up to a three-fold reduction in fertility following RPC for UC. One study used hysterosalpingography (HSG) to assess tubal morphology in 21 patients who had undergone RPC. Only 7 patients showed normal tubal anatomy, with 11 patients showing tubular occlusion and 10 having tubular adhesions. Another study reported that unresolved infertility problems were more common in patients treated surgically for IBD, and reported bilateral pelvic tubal adhesions in a small number of patients who had an ileal pouch. Fecundity rates in females undergoing ileo-rectal anastomosis are better than in females undergoing RPC. This suggests that RPC may affect fertility through more than one mechanism, as it would be expected that the operation of ileo-rectal anastomosis would also lead to pelvic adhesions. The additional pelvic dissection around the ovaries during the RPC may play a role in the reduction in fertility and could explain why there is less of a reduction in fertility in an ileo-rectal anastomosis. The reduction in the ability to conceive may be due to the formation of pelvic adhesions causing obstruction of the Fallopian tubes. The recognition of the significant effect of pelvic surgery, and RPC in particular, on fecundity have meant that this is an important pre-operative discussion in all women of childbearing age.

There have been varying reports on the incidence of fertility treatment use in females following RPC. A recent study from Finland retrospectively compared fertility and pregnancy of 138 RPC patients with 130 patients having had an appendicectomy. Fertility treatment was required in 24% and 10% of the patients, respectively. In another study however, there was no significant difference in the use of fertility treatments before and after RPC. In a study of 237 females, 30% of the children born to women following RPC were conceived using *in vitro* fertilization (IVF) compared with 1% in the general population. IVF treatment is potentially a treatment option for women following RPC, but this should be discussed with the relevant gynaecologist as there may be other factors involved.

Pregnancy and IBD

IBD peaks in incidence during patients' reproductive years. European incidences reported from a large multicentre epidemiological study for UC and CD are 10.4/100,000 and 5.6/100,000 per year, respectively. Opinion on the effect of IBD on pregnancy is varied, with a number of studies reporting that IBD does not have an adverse effect on the outcome of pregnancy. Several population-based case control studies have reported no increase in stillbirth, neonatal death, or spontaneous abortion. An association between IBD and premature births (<37 weeks) and low

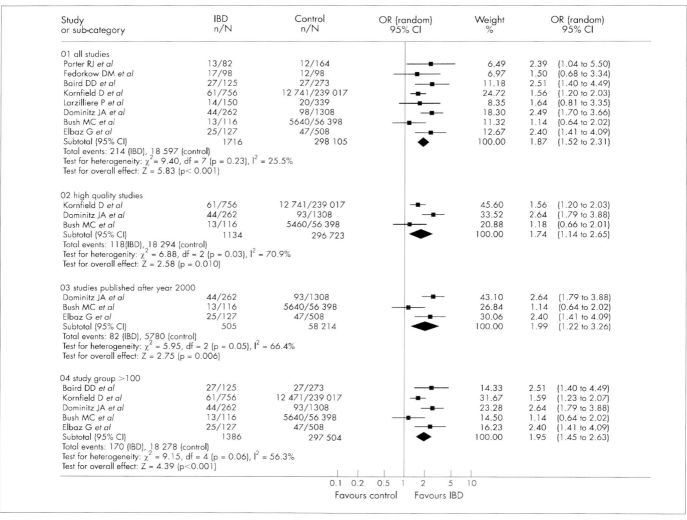

8.1 Forest plot demonstrating the risk of prematurity in the IBD population *vs.* the general population. (From Cornish J, Tan E, Teare J, *et al.* A meta-analysis on the influence of inflammatory bowel disease on pregnancy. *Gut* 2007;**56**(6):830–7.)

birth weight infants (<2,500 g) has been described.

The results of a recent meta-analysis, with 3,907 IBD patients and 320,531 controls, suggests that women with IBD were more likely to suffer adverse pregnancy outcomes, in particular premature birth, low birth weight, and undergo a Caesarean section. Patients with IBD were nearly twice as likely to have a premature delivery (<37 weeks' gestation) compard to the normal population, a result which remained significant after the sensitivity analysis (**8.1**).

Females with UC have a higher risk of a foetus with congenital abnormalities than the general population (odds ratio 3.88). It was reported that females with IBD have a 1.5-fold risk of a Caesarean section compared to the general population (**8.2**).

There was no significant difference in premature birth between patients with CD or UC. The impact of premature delivery on an infant's physical, mental, and social health may be substantial and women with IBD must be aware of increased risk of prematurity in their babies.

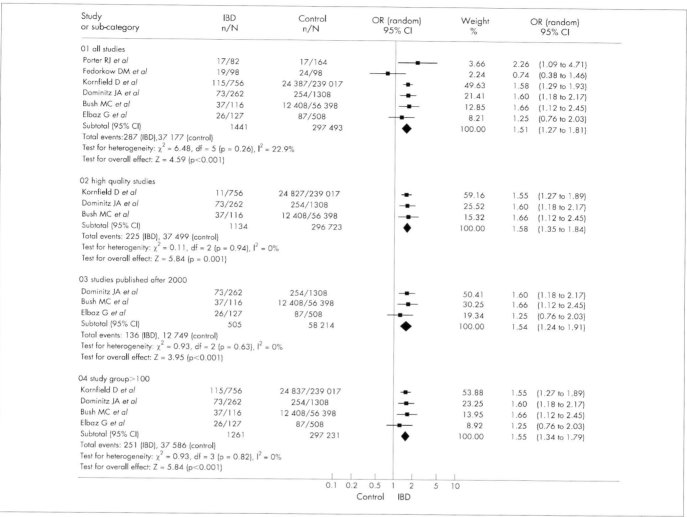

8.2 Comparison of the risk of Caesarean section in females with IBD *vs.* the general population. (From Cornish J, Tan E, Teare J, *et al.* A meta-analysis on the influence of inflammatory bowel disease on pregnancy. *Gut* 2007;**56**(6):830–7.)

Pregnancy and restorative proctocolectomy

Three studies of 423 patients did not demonstrate an increase in the incidence of complications during pregnancy following RPC. The incidence of pre-eclampsia (3%) and gestational diabetes (1%) in patients who underwent RPC was less than that of the general population, as was the incidence of miscarriage and stillbirths. Pouch function during pregnancy has been shown to change significantly, with an increase being reported in stool frequency, incontinence, and pad usage. This is particularly seen in the third trimester of pregnancy. Post-partum, the pouch function appears to return to the pre-pregnancy state, usually within 6 months. It has been suggested by Hahnloser *et al*. that pouch function then deteriorates over time, with daytime stool frequency being increased at the time of their last follow-up, 68 months after delivery (median daytime stool frequency 5.4 *vs*. 6.4; p <0.001).

There is evidence from several studies that vaginal delivery is not contra-indicated following RPC. Care must be taken however, as although short-term follow-up of bowel function and continence suggests that vaginal delivery does not have an adverse impact, it can be seen in a study by Polle *et al*. that women who have a complicated vaginal delivery following RPC have a higher risk of incontinence with ageing and long-term follow-up. The method of delivery should be dictated by obstetric considerations in the majority of patients, although Caesarean section is recommended for those patients with a scarred and rigid perineum.

Medications during pregnancy

Management of pregnancies in women with IBD can be difficult in a variety of aspects of treatment. Controlling remission of the disease prior to and during conception is important for the health of the foetus and the mother. If a woman conceives while her disease is active, she is more likely to have a premature or low birth weight infant than a woman who has quiescent disease. The incidence of stillbirths and spontaneous abortions is also related to disease activity. The frequency of relapses is no greater if pregnant, and if relapses do occur they tend to do so in the first trimester of pregnancy.

A review of nineteen studies, with 1,962 women, reported that the use of corticosteroids for IBD during pregnancy was not associated with an increase in stillbirth, ectopic pregnancies, spontaneous abortions, or low birth weight infants (*Table 8.1*). Aza was associated with a higher risk of

Table 8.1 Pregnancy outcomes and medications for IBD

Outcomes	5-ASA	Azathioprine	Corticosteroids	Anti-TNF-	Normal population incidence
No. of studies	14	3	4	6	
No. of women	1,026	37	883	110	
No. of pregnancies	648	39	581	95	
No. of successful pregnancies	94% (612)	85% (33)	94% (546)	72% (68)	
Spontaneous abortion	2.4% (16)	3% (1)	<1% (2)	16% (11)	20%
Elective termination	1% (7)	6% (2)	0	24% (16)	0.02%
Stillbirths	<1% (4)	0	<1% (1)	0	<1%
LBW	<1% (4)	3% (1)	3% (4)	3% (2)	7.6%
Premature birth	1% (7)	15% (5)	2% (3)	9% (6)	
Ectopic pregnancy	<1% (1)	0	0	0	1%
Major congenital defect	1.6% (10)	6% (2)	11% (14)	3% (2)	<1%

major congenital defects than in the general population (6% Aza *vs.* <1% for general population), but no increase in other adverse events during pregnancy. The comparison with the general IBD population is not known and it is generally recommended that Aza should be continued in pregnancy, particularly if the disease has previously been difficult to control. 5-ASA medications were not associated with an increase in stillbirth, ectopic pregnancies, spontaneous abortions, or low birth weight infants. Anti-TNF-α drugs during pregnancy have not been demonstrated to have an incidence of adverse events during pregnancy. A significantly higher rate of therapeutic terminations has been reported for patients on the medication during pregnancy compared with the general population (19% *vs.* 0.02%). Methotrexate is contraindicated during pregnancy due to its teratogenic properties.

In view of the increased risk of adverse pregnancy outcomes with active disease, the management of pregnancy in IBD patients needs to focus on maintaining disease remission prior to and during pregnancy. Patients and their partners should be involved very early in the pregnancy or ideally while planning a family. Close interaction between the obstetrician and gastroenterologist and the couple is essential for best management and compliance. Many women may feel that they do not want to take any medications during a pregnancy. This initial reaction should be respected, but for patients who have difficulty in control it is important that they are aware of the risks of not controlling their disease. Equally, women and their partners should be aware of any adverse pregnancy outcomes associated with the medication they are taking. Counselling is advised and should be offered to minimize difficulties for the couple and the clinicians dealing with them during the pregnancy.

Recommended reading

Alstead EM, Ritchie JK, Lennard-Jones JE, Farthing MJ, Clark ML. Safety of azathioprine in pregnancy in inflammatory bowel disease. *Gastroenterology* 1990;**99**:443–6.

Alstead EM, Nelson-Piercy C. Inflammatory bowel disease in pregnancy. *Gut* 2003;**52**:159–61.

Baird DD, Narendranathan M, Sandler RS. Increased risk of preterm birth for women with inflammatory bowel disease. *Gastroenterology* 1990;**99**:987–94.

Cornish JA, Tan E, Teare J, *et al.* The effect of restorative proctocolectomy on sexual function, urinary function, fertility, pregnancy and delivery: A systematic review. *Dis Colon Rectum* 2007;**50**:1128–38.

Friedman S. Management of inflammatory bowel disease during pregnancy and nursing. *Semin Gastrointest Dis* 2001;**12**:245–52.

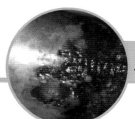

Chapter 9

Extraintestinal manifestations

Introduction

Both UC and CD may be complicated by inflammation outside the GI tract. Almost every organ system has been implicated at some time (*Table 9.1*); however, by far the commonest systems to be affected are the joints, skin, eyes, and liver. Interestingly while some manifestations are clearly associated with active intestinal inflammation a number of them appear to run a course independent of the bowel disease. The relationship with the bowel disease is listed in *Table 9.2*.

Table 9.1 Extraintesinal manifestations reported in IBD

Musculoskeletal
Peripheral arthritis
Granulomatous arthritis and
  synovitis
Rheumatoid arthritis
Sacroiliitis
Ankylosing spondylitis
Clubbing
Osteoporosis and
  osteomalacia
Rhabdomyolysis
Relapsing polychondritis

***Skin and mucous
membranes***
Oral ulceraton
Cheilitis
Pyostomatitis vegetans
Erythema nodosum
Sweet's syndrome
Metastatic CD
Psoriasis
Epidermolysis bullosa
  acquisita

Perianal skin tags
Polyarteritis nodosa
Cutaneous vasculitis

Neurologic
Peripheral neuropathy
Meningitis
Vestibular dysfunction
Pseudotumour cerebri

Ocular
Conjunctivitis
Uveitis, iritis
Episcleritis
Scleritis
Retrobulbar neuritis
Crohn's keratopathy

Bronchopulmonary
Chronic bronchitis with
  bronchiectasis
Fibrosing alveolitis
Pulmonary vasculitis
Interstitial lung disease

Sarcoidosis
Tracheal obstruction

Cardiac
Pleuropericarditis
Cardiomyopathy
Endocarditis
Myocarditis

Endocrine and metabolic
Growth failure
Thyroiditis
Osteoporosis, osteomalacia

Haematologic
Anaemia – iron deficiency
Vitamin B12 deficiency
Anaemia of chronic diseases
Autoimmune haemolytic
  anaemia
Hyposplenism
Anticardiolipin antibody
Takayasu's arteritis

Wegener's arteritis

Renal and genitourinary
Nephrolithiasis
Retroperitoneal fibrosis
Fistula formation
Glomerulonephritis
Renal amyloidosis
Drug-related nephrotoxicity

Hepatopancreatobiliary
Primary sclerosing
  cholangitis (PSC)
Small duct PSC
Cholangiocarcinoma
Cholelithiasis
Autoimmune hepatitis
Primary biliary cirrhosis
Pancreatitis
Ampullary CD
Granulomatous pancreatitis

Table 9.2 Relationship between extraintestinal manifestations (EIMs) and bowel disease activity

EIMs associated with active disease	Type 1 (large joint) arthritis
	Erythema nodosum
	Ocular inflammation
	Pyoderma gangrenosum (sometimes)
EIMs not associated with active disease	Type 2 (small joint) arthritis
	Ankylosing spondylitis
	Pyoderma gangrenosum (usually)
	Primary sclerosing cholangitis

Arthritis

Either the axial skeleton or peripheral joints may be affected. Axial disease may take the form of ankylosing spondylitis (AS) or isolated sacroiliitis.

AS is a well characterized clinical syndrome consisting of sacroiliitis associated with signs and symptoms of progressive axial inflammation. These are listed in *Table 9.3*. It affects 1–6% of IBD patients, and unlike idiopathic AS affects men and women equally. The progressive nature of the disease leads to immobility of the spine, and fusion of the vertebral facet joints means that patients adopt a characteristic 'question mark' posture (**9.1**). Other complications such as respiratory embarrassment and upper lobe lung fibrosis as a result of fusion of the ribs may also occur. The spinal disease may present before or after the gut disease and runs a course independent of the bowel. As with idiopathic AS it is associated with possession of HLA-B27, but the association is less strong, with only 50–70% of patients possessing it compared to over 90% in idiopathic AS. Possible treatment modalities for AS are summarized in *Table 9.4*. The mainstay of treatment is effective physical therapy with exercises to improve spinal mobility. Drug treatment begins initially with analgesics and anti-inflammatory drugs, but NSAID use runs the risk of exacerbating the underlying IBD. Sulfasalazine may be used, but is largely ineffective on the axial disease, as is methotrexate. In patients with persistent stiffness and immobility the advent of anti-TNF therapy has made a big impact, and may treat both the axial skeletal disease and the underlying gut disease, although there is little evidence to

Table 9.3 Clinical features of ankylosing spondylitis

Sacroiliitis

Inflammatory back pain and immobility

Enthesitis

Respiratory embarrassment

Aortic root problems

Peripheral arthritis in 30%

Uveitis in 20–40%

suggest that even this therapy has a major impact on the long-term outlook for the axial disease.

Isolated sacroiliitis is much more common that AS, but rarely causes significant symptoms. It may be found in up to 30% of UC patients and 40% of CD patients, and is often an incidental finding on a plain abdominal radiograph. It does not appear to have an association with HLA-B27, and it is not clear which of these patients progress to develop full blown AS. Patients who have symptoms of inflammatory low back pain (*Table 9.5*) should be given advice about spinal exercises, and should have their spinal mobility checked regularly to make sure there are no signs of progressive disease which may need more aggressive treatment. A positive HLA-B27 test may give a higher index of suspicion for progressive disease and may therefore be useful in this context.

Table 9.4 Treatment options for ankylosing spondylitis

Physical therapy	Spinal mobility exercises to maintain spinal flexibility
Analgesia	Simple analgesia NSAIDs if bowel disease quiescent
Local therapy	Intra-articular steroid injection (short-lived benefit only)
Immune modulators	Oral prednisolone (short-term relief) Methotrexate (more effective for peripheral joint disease)
Biological therapy	Adalimumab or infliximab – treat both joints and gut Etanercept – effective for joints but not gut

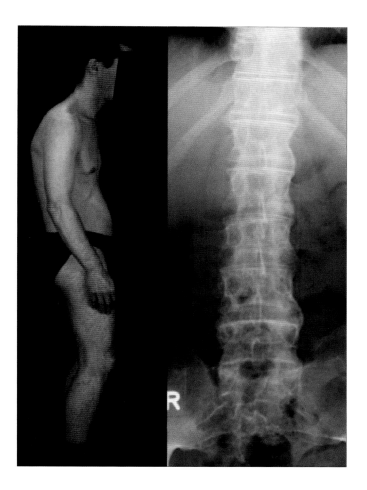

Table 9.5 Clinical features distinguishing inflammatory and mechanical low back pain

Mechanical back pain

Gets worse as the day goes on

Improves with rest

Inflammatory back pain

Worse in the morning

Associated with morning stiffness >30 mins

Improves with exercise

Radiates into the buttocks

Impairs spinal flexion

9.1 The 'question mark' posture of ankylosing spondylitis, with the corresponding radiological appearance of a bamboo spine. (Courtesy of Prof. Peter Taylor, Kennedy Institute of Rheumatology, Imperial College London.)

Peripheral arthritis

This is the commonest extraintestinal manifestation of IBD, with 20–30% of patients suffering at some stage in their disease from an inflammatory arthropathy. There are two forms of peripheral arthritis seen in IBD, summarized in *Table 9.6*. Type 1 is associated with active intestinal inflammation, and is very similar to the reactive arthritis seen after gut or genitourinary infections, whereas Type 2 is a more persistent polyarthritis. It is important to note that neither form of arthropathy is erosive or deforming, and in patients with erosive arthritis another diagnosis should be considered such as rheumatoid or psoriatic arthritis.

Treatment of Type 1 arthritis is normally that of the underlying gut disease, as when this is under control the joints normally settle. However, in the short term intra-articular steroid injection may help symptomatically along with simple analgesia. NSAIDs should be avoided. For more persistent arthritis occasionally specific treatment of the arthritis is required, and this may include low-dose steroids or immune suppressants such as methotrexate. Occasionally biological therapy such as infliximab may be required, and has been reported as effective.

Table 9.6 Forms of peripheral arthritis in IBD

Type 1 (pauciarticular)

Fewer than 5 joints, always including a large joint

Self-limiting episodes often with relapses of IBD

Associated with HLA B*27 and DRB1*0103

Type 2 (polyarticular)

More than 5 joints often involving small joints, especially MCP

Persistent symptoms running a course independent of the IBD

Skin manifestations

The commonest skin manifestation of IBD is erythema nodosum. Pyoderma gangrenosum is less common but can cause major problems for the patient.

Erythema nodosum

Erythema nodosum (EN) is a painful raised erythematous rash with characteristic raised, tender nodules which particularly affect the extensor surfaces of the lower extremities (**9.2**). It occurs in up to 15% of CD patients, but is much less common in UC; there is a large female preponderance, with a F:M ratio of 5:1. In the vast majority of cases (>90%) it occurs in conjunction with active bowel disease.

The aetiology of EN in IBD remains uncertain, but intriguingly there appears to be a genetic rearrangement at the HLA-B locus, with several rare alleles being more common than expected.

As the lesions are typically associated with an exacerbation of the IBD, treatment is mainly directed towards the underlying disease; indeed in a study including 48 patients with EN, all responded to the IBD treatment. Symptomatic relief may be gained by the elevation of an affected limb; as discussed above, NSAIDs should be used as analgesia only with extreme caution in the context of active bowel disease. In refractory cases, potassium iodide, systemic corticosteroids, colchicine, hydroxychloroquine, and infliximab have been used with some success.

Pyoderma gangrenosum

Pyoderma gangrenosum (PG) is a much rarer EIM, with a prevalence of 0.4–2%. Initial discrete pustules or fluctuant nodules evolve into ulcerating lesions with undermined, violaceous edges and surrounding erythema (**9.3**). They commonly occur on the shins or adjacent to stomas, but can manifest anywhere on the body. The diagnosis is made on clinical grounds, though wound swabs and a skin biopsy may be needed to exclude other conditions.

A small study has recently shown that patients with IBD-associated PG are more likely to suffer from the other musculoskeletal, ocular, and mucocutaneous EIMs, and has found an increased prevalence of HLA DRB1*0103 in these patients. PG may run a course independent of the IBD, but treatment should be aimed at both. Given its rarity, there have been few controlled trials investigating the treatment of PG. Some authorities advocate gentle debridement of the ulcer but most are of the opinion that this can make matters worse as the lesions exhibit pathergy – they can be induced or extended by trauma. For this reason, aggressive surgical debridement or skin grafting is discouraged, though occasionally it may be used in patients with remitting or stable disease in conjunction with immune suppressants.

Topical and intralesional corticosteroids have been employed, as have topical 5-ASA and sodium cromoglycate. Systemic therapy is usually required however, and prednisolone is considered the first-line drug of choice.

Other systemic agents used include oral ciclosporin and tacrolimus, though recent trial data have suggested that infliximab may be the drug of choice in refractory cases, probably in conjunction with another immunosuppressant such as Aza.

Rare skin manifestations are listed in *Table 9.1*: Sweet's syndrome is an acute febrile neutrophilic dermatosis, and patients present with a fever, leucocytosis, and raised ESR, with a characteristic vesicular rash. It usually responds well to steroid therapy.

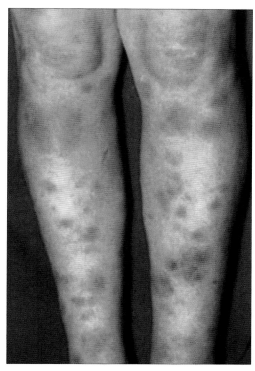

9.2 The typical rash of erythema nodosum.

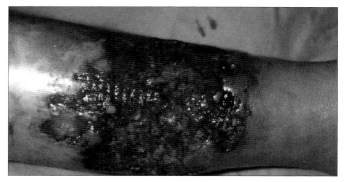

9.3 Pyoderma gangrenosum – this exhibits the classical appearance of violaceous overhung edges.

Ocular manifestations

The prevalence of ocular inflammation in IBD is less than 10%, but its prompt recognition is vital. It may result in significant morbidity, including blindness, and referral to an ophthalmologist for a thorough evaluation is recommended.

Episcleritis
The most common ocular complication is episcleritis, presenting with redness of one or both eyes and a sensation of irritation but no visual loss. Episcleritis often parallels the underlying IBD and usually responds to treatment of the gut disease. Specific treatment may include topical steroids; oral NSAIDs are often effective but, as discussed above, should be used with great caution in active IBD.

Scleritis
Scleritis is a more serious condition which may lead to impairment of vision, and can result in retinal detachment. It typically presents with severe pain and tenderness to palpation. Management is with systemic steroids, NSAIDs, or immunosuppressants.

Uveitis
Uveitis, a condition associated with HLA-B*27, B*58, and HLA-DRB1*0103 in IBD, often occurs independently of the bowel disease and is particularly associated with the musculoskeletal EIMs. It presents with a painful red eye, photophobia, and blurred vision. Treatment involves the use of cycloplegics and topical steroids though systemic steroids or immunosuppression are often required.

In the management of ocular inflammation, sulfasalazine, methotrexate, and mycophenolate mofetil have all been trialled with some success. Infliximab is increasingly being used in both acute and chronic ocular inflammatory conditions though trials have, to date, been small.

Liver disease

Primary sclerosing cholangitis (PSC)
PSC is a chronic progressive cholestatic liver disease which is associated with IBD in approximately two-thirds of cases. The diagnosis is often made in asymptomatic patients with abnormal liver function tests noted in routine follow-up. If symptomatic, patients may complain of fatigue, itching, fever, right upper quadrant pain, and weight loss.

Increasingly, noninvasive magnetic resonance cholangiopancreatography (MRCP) is used for diagnosis in preference to the traditional gold standard, endoscopic retrograde cholangiopancreatography (ERCP). It has been suggested that ERCP should remain the confirmatory test given its higher specificity or should perhaps be reserved for patients in whom the diagnosis is uncertain after MRCP. Liver biopsy rather than ERCP may be the favoured approach if an MRCP is negative and the index of suspicion is low. If performed, typical features at liver biopsy are periductal inflammation and fibrosis, bile ductular proliferation, and portal tract inflammation (**9.4**).

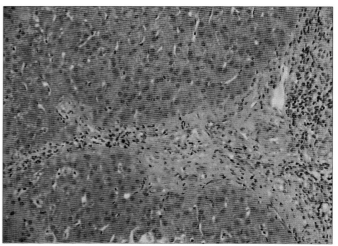

9.4 Primary sclerosing cholangitis in a patient with ulcerative colitis, with periductal inflammation and fibrosis.

Medical and endoscopic management

Ursodeoxycholic acid (UDCA) has been extensively studied in the treatment of PSC and is widely prescribed for this indication. The largest trial of UDCA, at lower doses of 13–15 mg/kg, found improvements in liver biochemistry but not histology. Recent studies have shown that biliary enrichment in PSC increases with increasing dose, and plateaus at 22–25 mg/kg. Significant effects on progression of cholangiographic appearances and liver fibrosis were found in a trial using high doses. The largest trial to date using high doses showed a nonsignificant trend towards improved survival and reduced need for liver transplantation; histological progression was not assessed.

Steroids have not been shown to benefit PSC patients, and trials of immune suppressants have not demonstrated consistent benefits. Tight strictures in the biliary tree can be treated endoscopically with balloon dilatation or biliary stents.

Cholangiocarcinoma and colonic carcinoma

Cholangiocarcinoma will develop in approximately 10–30% of patients with PSC, but to date there are no reliable means of identifying those at particular risk. There are data to suggest that UDCA treatment may have a chemopreventive effect against cholangiocarcinoma.

PSC patients are also at particularly high risk of colonic dysplasia and cancer and it is recommended that those with UC undergo yearly surveillance colonoscopy. As with cholangiocarcinoma, there is evidence that UDCA may have a role in preventing colonic neoplasia. In the largest series reported, a small reduction in colonic dysplasia and cancer was found, not reaching significance; other studies, however, have demonstrated significant reductions.

Liver transplantation

In advanced PSC, orthotopic liver transplantation remains the only treatment of proven benefit, with a 5-year survival of roughly 70%. PSC recurs in 20–40% of recipients.

Recommended reading

Williams H, Walker D, Orchard TR. Extraintestinal manifestations of inflammatory bowel disease. *Curr Gastroenterol Rep* 2008 Dec;**10**(6):597–605.

Orchard TR, Thiyagaraja S, Welsh KI, Wordsworth BP, Hill Gaston JS, Jewell DP. Clinical phenotype is related to HLA genotype in the peripheral arthropathies of inflammatory bowel disease. *Gastroenterology* 2000 Feb;**118**(2):274–8.

Orchard TR, Chua CN, Ahmad T, Cheng H, Welsh KI, Jewell DP. Uveitis and erythema nodosum in inflammatory bowel disease: clinical features and the role of HLA genes. *Gastroenterology* 2002 Sep;**123**(3):714–18.

Chapter 10

Malignancy in inflammatory bowel disease

Colon cancer

One of the most concerning complications of IBD is the development of colon cancer. The overall mortality of IBD has dramatically reduced in the last 50 years, but there remains a small excess of deaths that are largely due to the long-term development of malignant complications. It was originally thought that the risk was largely restricted to UC, but it is now generally accepted that patients with extensive colonic involvement with CD are also at higher risk. The groups thought to be at highest risk are listed in *Table 10.1*. Patients with a long history of extensive colonic disease are at highest risk, particularly those with persistent or recurrent inflammation. The risk begins to increase substantially approximately 8 years after the beginning of the disease, and thus most surveillance programmes begin at this stage. Most of the risk factors could be considered to reflect the 'dose' of inflammatory burden that the colonic epithelium is exposed to over time. Data from St Mark's Hospital in London have also correlated persistent colonic inflammation observed during colonoscopic surveillance with an increased risk of colo-rectal cancer (CRC). Conversely, patients without evidence of persistent inflammation have a cancer risk equivalent to that of the background population. CRC is believed to arise from dysplastic epithelium within the colonic mucosa, and in turn dysplasia is thought to be driven by persistent mucosal inflammation. The inflammatory milieu present in the inflamed colonic mucosa is characterized by the presence of pro-inflammatory cytokines and the generation of reactive oxygen species and other mediators that can directly damage deoxyribonucleic acid (DNA). In the presence of chronic inflammation and tissue injury there is also local generation of growth factors and other signals that promote and propagate cellular proliferation in an attempt to repair the injured mucosa. It is easy to envisage theoretically how neoplastic changes might be inclined to evolve when DNA damage occurs in the context of strong stimuli for cellular proliferation. Some commentators have described this hypothesis as the chronic inflammation–dysplasia–carcinoma sequence.

One other specific group of patients at risk of developing colon cancer appears to be patients with PSC. Interestingly these patients may have disease which appears clinically quite quiescent, while having a very substantial increase in risk. This may be because the disease is normally a pancolitis (sometimes with rectal sparing) and endoscopic appearances often suggest more severe disease than suggested by the clinical features.

Table 10.1 Risk factors for developing colorectal cancer

Disease duration >8 years

Extensive disease (beyond the splenic flexure)

Recurrent or persistent inflammation

Coexisting primary sclerosing cholangitis (PSC)

The degree of elevation in the risk of colon cancer is a matter of some debate. Early studies suggested that the rate of colon cancer development was very substantial, peaking at about the age of 50 years, and increasing proportionately to the length of the disease history (**10.1**). Subsequent studies have suggested that the rates may be rather lower. The results of two large studies are recorded in *Table 10.2*. Both have lower rates than the early studies, probably due to the widespread use of 5-ASA (see below), but in addition the Danish study was conducted in a centre with a low threshold for colectomy (which will largely remove the cancer risk), and this may account for the relatively lower rate.

It is important to remember that while a panprocto-colectomy and end-ileostomy will effectively remove any risk of colon cancer, operations such as the formation of an ileo-anal pouch may leave a small segment of rectum *in situ* in which malignant change may occur; this may need to be surveyed regularly with a rigid sigmoidoscope in order to minimize the small risk of malignant transformation.

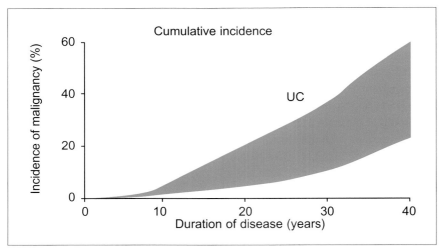

10.1 The incidence of UC with time after diagnosis.

Table 10.2 Cancer risk in UC – UK and Danish studies (Eaden 2001 and Winther)

	Prevalence of CRC (%)	
Length of history	*UK study (Eaden)*	*Danish study (Winther)*
Overall	3.7 (5.4 in pancolitis)	
10 years	2	0.2
20 years	8	1.4
30 years	18	3.1

Interventions to minimize risk

Prevention

There has been increasing interest in the role of 5-ASA medications as possible chemopreventative agents in preventing colon cancer in UC. The difficulty in trying to assess their effectiveness lies in the fact that they are so widely used as maintenance therapy for UC that it would not be ethical to do a placebo-controlled study to measure this effect formally. Thus data are derived from retrospective studies and meta-analyses. These suggest that patients who take 5-ASA daily as maintenance therapy experience a substantial risk reduction of between 50 and 80%. In one study, patients who took more than 1.2 g daily experienced a risk reduction of over 90%. It is difficult to know how this effect is mediated, but one possible explanation is via a cellular nuclear receptor, PPARγ. This receptor controls the expression of a large number of regulatory genes, and is normally highly expressed in colonic epithelium; however, it is expressed at decreased levels in UC. PPARγ has also been implicated in adenocarcinogenesis in mouse models, where the addition of topical 5-ASA has reduced tumour size by up to 80%; an effect blocked by a competitive PPARγ inhibitor. Thus there appears to be at least one plausible biological mechanism for the action of 5-ASA in preventing the development of cancer in UC.

In patients with PSC it is possible that regular UDCA may have an additive effect on reducing the risk of colon cancer, but the mechanism of this remains unknown.

Surveillance

The increased risk of colorectal cancer in UC has meant that most countries have guidelines suggesting colonoscopic surveillance in high risk patients. Two sets of guidelines that are widely used are those of the American Society of Gastrointestinal Endoscopy (ASGE) and those of the British Society of Gastroenterology (BSG).

Both sets of guidelines suggest beginning colonoscopic surveillance 8–10 years after diagnosis, and then to continue thereafter depending on the findings. The ASGE guidelines suggest that patients with extensive disease should undergo colonoscopy every 1–2 years with random biopsies taken every 10 cm of the affected gut. For patients with left-sided disease (but proximal to the rectum) the ASGE guidelines suggest beginning surveillance at 15 years.

The recent BSG guidelines are based upon a number of studies that demonstrate that cancer risk is related to disease activity as well as extent, and that patients with a normal colonoscopy at 8–10 years have a very low risk of developing colorectal cancer. The converse is also true in that patients with evidence of significant inflammatory activity have a higher risk. Thus the recommended intervals vary according to the findings at the colonoscopy 8–10 years after diagnosis, and are shown in Figure 10.2. In addition, the guidelines take account of studies which demonstrate that dysplastic lesions can be usually be identified by chromoendoscopy (coating the colonic mucosa with dye-spray, such as indigo carmine). Thus the BSG guidelines suggest that, ideally, targeted biopsies should be taken from abnormal areas identified by chromoendoscopy. If chromoendoscopy is not available then a more traditional set of random biopsies every 10 cm should be taken.

Endoscopically visible lesions that are associated with an increased risk of dysplasia include strictures, raised lesions, depressed lesions, mucosal irregularity, inflammatory pseudopolyps, and areas of severe inflammation. This heterogeneous mixture of mucosal lesions termed DALMs (dysplasia-associated lesions/masses). Pseudopolyps may present particular difficulties, as the detection of dysplastic lesions in these areas can be particularly problematic, especially in the presence of active inflammation (10.3, 10.4). In addition to these, lesions resembling sporadic adenomas may also occur in patients with IBD and are termed ALMs (adenoma-like dysplastic lesions or mass). It is important to distinguish between these two types of lesion as the management is very different. Therefore, in addition to random biopsies, focused biopsies targeting specific mucosal abnormalities, including DALMs and ALMs are also necessary. When specific lesions are targeted, biopsies from the surrounding mucosa are also sampled to detect any 'flat' areas of dysplasia outside of the visible lesion. The finding of dysplasia within a DALM or within the background mucosa is an indication for colectomy; however, if dysplasia is confined to an ALM there is increasing evidence that these lesions can be treated like sporadic adenomas in the general population, with polypectomy and surveillance.

Sometimes distinguishing between DALMs and sporadic adenomas can be difficult and management decisions in these patients should involve honest and open discussions with the patient. Options include polypectomy followed by

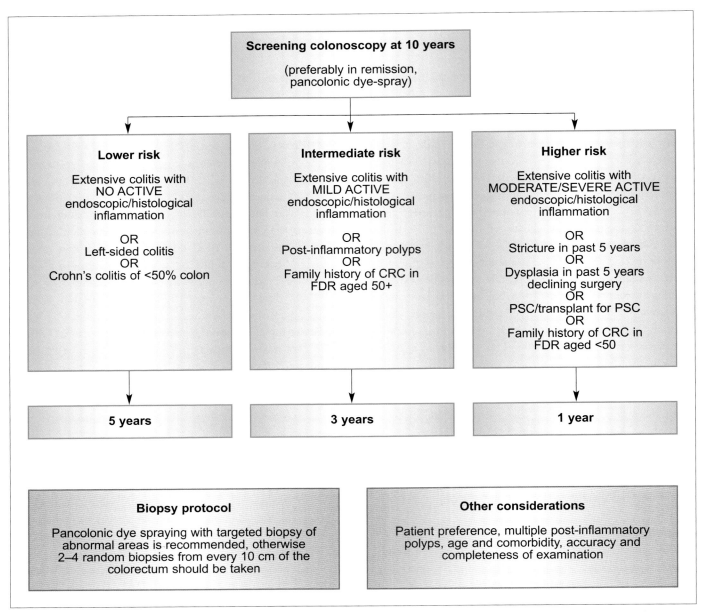

10.2 Current recommendations from the BSG for surveillance colonoscopy in UC. CRC, colorectal cancer; FDR, first degree relative; PSC, primary sclerosing cholangitis. (Adapted from Cairns SR *et al*. Guidleines for colorectal cancer screening and surveillance in moderate and high risk groups (update from 2002). *Gut* 2010;**59**:666–90.)

more intensive surveillance (e.g. 3-monthly colonoscopy) or consideration of immediate colectomy. Lesions resembling sporadic adenomas arising in areas of prominent inflammatory change should be regarded with particular suspicion and a lower threshold for recommending colectomy should be adopted.

The detection of 'high-grade' dysplasia (corroborated by two independent histopathologists) in random colonic biopsies, or within DALMs following surveillance colonoscopy in IBD, is an indication for colectomy. More than half of patients with 'high-grade' dysplasia will have evidence of CRC within the colectomy specimen. However, the management of 'low-grade' dysplasia is more controversial. Data from the St Mark's Hospital surveillance

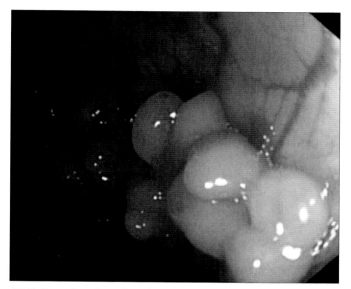

10.3 Pseudopolyps forming a mass on a background of quiescent UC.

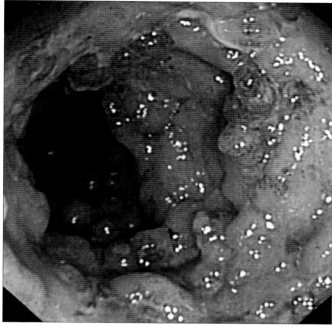

10.4 Pseudopolyps on a background of active inflammation making detection of areas of dysplasia very difficult.

programme indicate that half of the patients with definite low-grade dysplasia will evolve to high-grade dysplasia or CRC within 5 years. Consequently, immediate colectomy in this setting is advocated by many clinicians and should probably be considered mandatory in patients with multifocal areas of low-grade dysplasia arising from flat mucosa. However, some would advocate a more intensive form of colonoscopic screening for patients with an isolated area of low-grade dysplasia.

Use of methylene blue or indigo carmine dye spray techniques (chromoendoscopy) can enhance mucosal views to such an extent that targeted biopsies of suspicious lesions can be taken without the requirement for routine random biopsies, hence their incorporation into the updated guidelines. Other new techniques such as narrow band imaging (NBI) require further evaluation before their routine use can be recommended, but may allow easier detection of dysplastic lesions (**10.5, 10.6**). An algorithm for the management of patients depending on the results of biopsies at colonoscopy is shown in Figure **10.7**. The evidence base for surveillance in colonic CD is less strong, but in general similar protocols to those for UC are recommended.

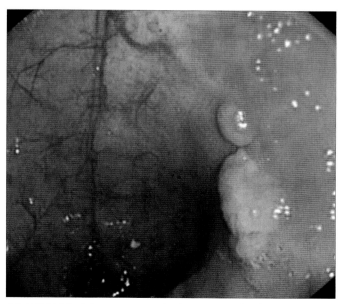

10.5 DALM at the upper end of an area of UC visible with white light colonoscopy.

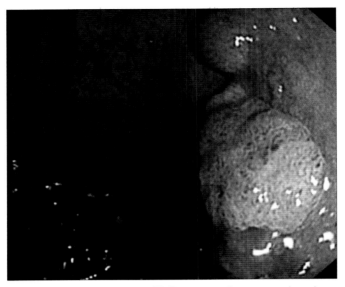

10.6 The same lesion as **10.5** seen under narrow band imaging (NBI).

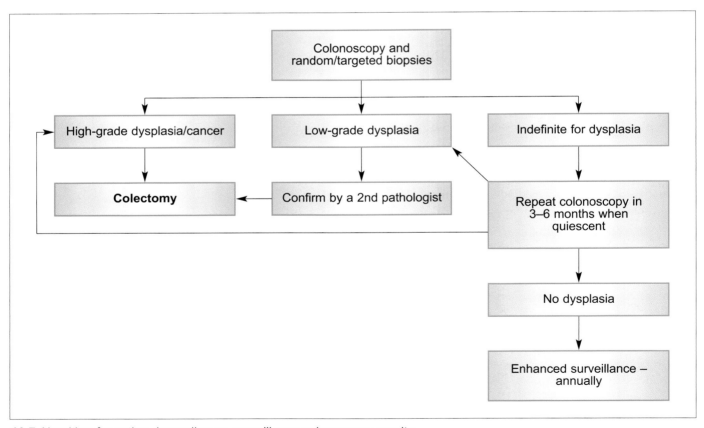

10.7 Algorithm for action depending on surveillance colonoscopy results.

Colectomy

Colectomy may be performed in patients identified by the surveillance programme or in special circumstances. The detection of high-grade dysplasia (corroborated by two independent histopathologists) in random colonic biopsies, or within DALMs following surveillance colonoscopy in IBD, is an indication for colectomy. More than half of patients with high-grade dysplasia will have evidence of CRC within the colectomy specimen. There remains some debate over the correct course of action in patients with low-grade dysplasia. If it is confirmed by two independent expert pathologists then many would advocate colectomy on the grounds that in these cases there is likely to be high-grade dysplasia or invasive carcinoma somewhere within the colon, with 50% having a focus of cancer in one study. If there is active inflammation with regeneration then there may be cellular atypia without the presence of dysplasia, and under these circumstances it can be difficult to differentiate dysplasia from atypia. This is illustrated in Figures **10.8**, **10.9**. If there is the possibility of dysplasia, but this cannot be confirmed ('indefinite for dysplasia') then a more conservative approach may be adopted with early re-colonoscopy and biopsy before making a definitive decision.

In patients with PSC who require liver transplantation the possibility of prophylactic colectomy may be considered, as patients will need lifelong immune suppression, and are known to be at high risk of developing colorectal carcinoma. These decisions need to be made after careful consideration and discussion with the patient.

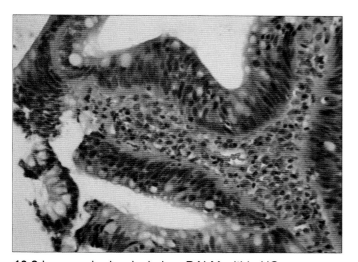

10.8 Low-grade dysplasia in a DALM within UC.

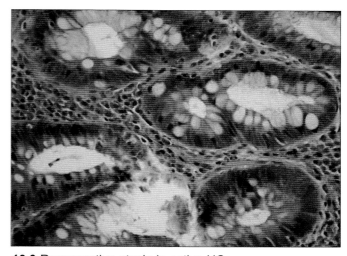

10.9 Regenerative atypia in active UC.

Other malignancies in IBD

Small bowel adenocarcinoma

There is a dramatically increased incidence of adeno-carcinoma of the small bowel in patients who suffer from small intestinal CD. This may be as much as 30 times the background rate. Despite this the frequency remains very small, and it remains much less common than adenocarcinoma of the colon.

Lymphomas

There is a small increase in the risk of lymphoma in CD compared to the background population, and this risk is mildly elevated further in patients who take immunosuppressive drugs such as Aza for long periods. If Aza is effective in a particular patient then the clinician and patient should have a discussion about whether to continue it in the long term after 2 or 3 years of therapy.

A very uncommon, but concerning association has been reported in CD patients concurrently treated with Aza and infliximab. This is the rare occurrence of hepatosplenic T cell lymphoma. This occurs generally in young people (aged 12–31 years) and is usually fatal. It is not known whether it is the particular combination of drugs and underlying disease that allows this to develop, but it does not seem to appear in the rheumatoid arthritis cohort of patients (possibly due to older age), and it is not clear whether other immune suppressants or anti-TNF therapies confer the same risk. However, in young patients it seems sensible to stop Aza a maximum of 6 months after starting treatment with biological therapy.

Drugs

As stated above, some drugs used in IBD may be associated with an increased risk of malignancy. It is difficult to know whether the new biological therapies are associated with an increased risk, as long-term safety data are not available. However, there are some case reports of patients developing solid organ and other tumours while on anti-TNF therapy, which have regressed dramatically upon ceasing it. Thus these treatments should be used with great care, particularly in those with a previous history of malignant disease.

PART III

OVERVIEW OF THERAPEUTIC MODALITIES IN INFLAMMATORY BOWEL DISEASE

Chapter 11
Drugs for inflammatory bowel disease

Introduction

Pharmacological therapy currently represents the mainstay of management of IBD. Broadly, the purpose of drug therapy in IBD can be simplified into three chief goals. Firstly, drugs are used to induce remission in patients with active, symptomatic disease, aiming to resolve symptoms and restore quality of life. Once in remission the second objective of drug therapy is to prevent relapse: IBD is typically a relapsing and remitting disease and drug-induced maintenance of long-term remission is a challenging objective. Some of the drugs employed in the management of IBD are capable of both inducing and maintaining clinical remission. The third goal of drug therapy is to prevent long-term complications of IBD, including surgeries and colorectal cancer.

The particular drug strategies employed are selected with these therapeutic goals in mind, but also on a number of other considerations such as disease severity, activity, and anatomical location. These variables dictate options such as route of administration (e.g. intravenous, oral, or rectally administered preparations such as suppositories or enemas), drug dosage, as well as the particular drug selected. For instance patients with mild UC are likely to respond to orally administered first-line agents such as aminosalicylates, whereas patients with more severe disease or with extensive disease are likely to need corticosteroids. Similarly, patients with isolated proctitis might respond better to rectally administered preparations such as suppositories where high dosages of active drug are delivered locally; whereas in patients with small bowel CD this approach would be clearly inappropriate. In addition to these general principles, clinicians should also focus on the extensive existing evidence base for specific drugs and therapeutic strategies in particular clinical settings.

Drugs employed in IBD are sometimes classified by mechanism of action, such as anti-inflammatories (corticosteroids and aminosalicylates) or immuno-modulators (Aza and methotrexate). In the last 10 years 'biological' therapies have emerged as exciting new treatment options in IBD. Biological therapies are engineered proteins that have been specifically developed for their high-affinity, specific interaction with mediators considered important in the inflammatory process. These drugs promise to revolutionize the pharmacological management of IBD. They also serve as an excellent paradigm of how an improved understanding of the molecular mechanisms that underpin particular disease states can lead to the development of specifically tailored therapeutic strategies.

Anti-inflammatory agents

Aminosalicylates

Sulfasalazine was the first widely available aminosalicylate drug. Like many drugs used in IBD, it was first used in the treatment of inflammatory arthritis. Most of the therapeutic benefit of sulfasalazine is believed to be derived from the 5-ASA component, which is chemically bound to a sulfapyridine carrier molecule. Following oral ingestion of sulfasalazine the azo bond linking the two components is lysed by colonic luminal bacteria, liberating the biologically active 5-ASA moiety. Although undoubtedly efficacious in the management of UC, sulfasalazine is associated with significant toxicity, ranging from relatively mild side-effects such as headache, rashes, nausea, and vomiting to serious adverse events such as Stevens–Johnson syndrome, agranulocytosis, pulmonary fibrosis, and male infertility (secondary to azoospermia), which is nearly always reversible upon stopping the drug. Most of the toxicity is due to the sulfapyridine moiety and consequently, new 'daughter' formulations of 5-ASA (also called mesalazine or mesalamine) drugs have been developed with alternative delivery systems, with the intention of retaining the clinical efficacy of sulfasalazine but improving the side-effect profile. Sulfasalazine is avoided by many clinicians, but in certain settings, such as troublesome articular manifestations complicating IBD, sulfasalazine is sometimes favoured in view of the long-term experience in treating rheumatoid arthritis.

Unfortunately, orally administered free, or unconjugated 5-ASA is rapidly absorbed in the jejunum and therapeutically active concentrations of drug fail to reach the distal small bowel or colon, where the majority of patients with CD and all patients with UC have disease. The new generation of 5-ASA compounds includes preparations that are specifically designed to release mesalazine in a time, pH, or luminal bacteria dependent fashion to ensure liberation of active mesalazine in the small intestine or colon. Commonly employed new generation preparations which deliver 5-ASA to the lower GI tract include Asacol® (Eudragit S coated), Salufalk® (Eudragit L coated), Pentasa® (coated microspheres), and Mesavant XL® (MMX) formulations of 5-ASA, olsalazine (two 5-ASA molecules bound together), and balsalazide (5-ASA attached to an inert carrier cleaved by colonic bacteria). The chemical structures and release mechanisms of these drugs are illustrated in Figure **11.1**.

In UC 5-ASAs have proven efficacy in both inducing

11.1 5-ASA compounds used in UC.

remission in patients with mild to moderate disease and also at maintaining remission. A Cochrane review performed in 2007 analysing data from eight randomized, placebo-controlled trials with over 1,000 patients reported that clinical remission or improvement could be achieved in 58% of patients with mild to moderate active UC treated with one of the new generation 5-ASAs compared to only 33% of placebo-treated patients. 5-ASAs are also effective at preventing disease relapse in patients with quiescent UC. Another Cochrane review (2006) reported a significantly reduced rate of clinical and endoscopic relapse in patients treated for at least 6 months with one of the new generation 5-ASA drugs, with a relapse rate of 50% in patients treated with 5-ASA compared to a relapse rate of 63% in placebo-treated patients. In patients with isolated distal disease, such as ulcerative proctitis, 5-ASA suppositories are at least as effective, if not better than, topical corticosteroids at both inducing and maintaining clinical remission. Even in patients with extensive UC (i.e. disease extending from the rectum to beyond the splenic flexure) of mild to moderate severity, the addition of 5-ASA enemas to standard oral 5-ASA treatment also significantly improves clinical response. There is also increasing evidence that dose escalation of 5-ASA (e.g. to >4 g per day) may also enhance clinical response, particularly with regard to speed of response. Patient compliance can be improved by reducing the dosing schedule to twice daily or once daily administration, rather than thrice daily administration: the latest addition to the 5-ASA armamentarium is a once daily dosing preparation that is encapsulated in a slow release multimatrix (MMX). This new formulation promises to prolong the exposure of 5-ASA to the colonic mucosa and allows high doses of 5-ASA to be taken in a single dose. Interestingly this may prove to be a class effect of 5-ASA rather than a feature of the MMX delivery system, as recent studies with other Eudragit and granular delivery systems (e.g. Pentasa and Salofalk) have demonstrated efficacy with once daily dosing.

The use of 5-ASAs in CD is more controversial, with conflicting reports regarding their capacity to either induce or maintain remission. However, their favourable side-effect profile without the need for intensive blood test monitoring, like that required for Aza for instance, means that some clinicians sometimes consider 5-ASA as a first-line therapy, particularly in clinical settings where they are felt to be potentially effective, such as in the prevention of post-operative recurrence. If 5-ASAs are to be considered in CD

they should preferably be administered in high doses (e.g. at least 4 g per day).

There is also mounting data to suggest that 5-ASAs may also reduce the risk of colorectal cancer in patients with long-standing UC or colonic CD (see Chapter 10, Malignancy in inflammatory bowel disease).

Corticosteroids

Corticosteroids have been routinely employed in the management of exacerbations of IBD since a ground-breaking placebo-controlled trial was published from Oxford in the 1950s demonstrating efficacy of cortisone in acute, severe colitis. A rapid clinical response can be expected in more than two-thirds of patients. In ambulant patients without severe disease, oral prednisolone 40 mg once daily, reducing by 5 mg per week, is a typical regime, although some centres, particularly in Europe, favour higher doses such as 1 mg/kg of body weight. Even in patients with mild to moderate disease, corticosteroids work faster and are more effective than 5-ASAs. Severe exacerbations, such as in patients with acute, severe colitis, should be admitted to hospital for intravenous corticosteroid therapy. Corticosteroid suppositories and liquid or foam enemas are available for patients with distal or left-sided disease, respectively. Although corticosteroids are extremely efficacious in bringing disease back into remission, they are not useful in maintaining remission of either UC or CD. Prolonged use of corticosteroids is also associated with significant toxicity, including osteoporosis, avascular necrosis, cataracts, obesity, acne, impaired glucose tolerance, and hypertension. New generation corticosteroids have been developed to try and improve the side-effect profile, and the most commonly employed in CD is budesonide. Budesonide is poorly absorbed from the GI tract and 90% of any drug absorbed is rapidly metabolized by the liver to limit potential systemic adverse effects. Budesonide formulations are available in coated preparations that lead to release of the active drug in the distal small bowel, generating maximal luminal concentrations of the active corticosteroid at the terminal ileum and right hemicolon. Such preparations are especially useful in patients with ileocolonic CD.

Immune suppressants (immunomodulators)

Immunodoulators are largely regarded as second-line agents in UC, but are extremely important in the management of CD, where the evidence base for using 5-ASA is clearly less robust. The most commonly employed immunomodulators are the purine analogue Aza, or its active metabolite 6-MP, and methotrexate.

Aza and 6-MP

Azathioprine is effective at both inducing and maintaining remission in both CD and UC. However, its slow onset of action (clinical response may take 12 weeks, and occasionally longer) usually limits its use as a first-line treatment in patients with active disease. It is most commonly employed in patients relapsing on 5-ASA treatment. UC patients experiencing repeated relapses despite taking 5-ASA maintenance therapy should be considered for Aza. In view of its slow onset of action Aza is often best started in patients experiencing disease flares who are treated initially with corticosteroids. As the corticosteroid dose is gradually withdrawn over 3 months, Aza is concomitantly prescribed with the intention of it becoming therapeutically active by the time the corticosteroids are finally stopped. Aza is administered orally and has a number of important side-effects, the most feared of which are myelosuppression, pancreatitis, and hepatitis. To counter these potential adverse effects, all patients taking Aza should have regular full blood counts and liver function test monitoring. Prior to starting Aza some clinicians advocate measuring the activity of the endogenous enzyme TPMT that is responsible for degrading Aza *in vivo*. The majority of the population has normal expression of TPMT and accordingly metabolizes Aza in a predictable fashion without accumulation of potentially toxic metabolites. However, 10% of the population have intermediate TPMT activity and about 0.3% have little or no TPMT activity. These patients are at much higher risk of developing myelosuppression or hepatitis and accordingly Aza dose is reduced, or the drug avoided in these patients. It is important to remember that testing for TPMT levels does not remove the necessity for regular blood monitoring in Aza treatment. Despite its predictive potential, the majority of patients who develop side-effects due to Aza have normal TPMT levels.

The choice between Aza and 6-MP is largely due to physician preference, although there is some evidence that 6-MP may have a better side-effect profile than Aza, and some patients who cannot tolerate Aza may tolerate 6-MP. Typical dosing would be Aza 2–2.5 mg/kg or 6-MP 1–1.5 mg/kg.

Methotrexate

Methotrexate is the second most commonly prescribed immunomodulator in IBD. There is good evidence from well conducted placebo-controlled trials that methotrexate is effective at both inducing and maintaining remission in CD. The best evidence is for once weekly intramuscular injection; however, some patients find this inconvenient and accordingly an oral preparation is also sometimes used. This may be from the date of commencing the drug, or patients may have 6 weeks of intramuscular therapy before being switched onto an oral preparation. There are few compelling data to support the use of methotrexate in UC, although retrospective series suggest that it may work in some patients intolerant of, or unresponsive to, Aza. Although immuno-modulator prescribing patterns are variable throughout Europe and the US, most clinicians would consider methotrexate in CD patients intolerant of thiopurines, and some would consider its use in UC. Side-effects from methotrexate may be severe, with mucositis, rashes, and dose-dependent hepatic fibrosis being the major problems. In addition, whereas Aza may be used with caution in pregnancy, methotrexate is contraindicated in patients who may become pregnant. The severe side-effects of methotrexate may be minimized by the administration of folic acid on one or more days when the methotrexate is not administered.

Other immune modulators

Ciclosporin has a major role as rescue therapy in patients with corticosteroid refractory acute, severe colitis (and which is discussed at length in Chapter 5, Acute, severe colitis). However, there is little evidence for its use orally in the long-term treatment of IBD. Other immunosuppressive drugs have not made it to mainstream clinical use in the management of IBD. There are numerous case reports, case series, and uncontrolled studies reporting the utility of tacrolimus, mycophenolate mofetil, and thalidomide in IBD, usually in patients with disease refractory to standard therapy. At present these agents should only be considered for use in specialist centres, mostly in the context of research.

Biological therapies

'Biological therapy' refers to a new class of therapeutic agents that threaten to revolutionize the management of IBD. These biosynthesized protein molecules are specifically designed to neutralize or antagonize mediators that are thought to be key components in the inflammatory processes that drive CD and UC. Typically these drugs are engineered from immunoglobulins, immunoglobulin fragments, or specific receptors because these molecules have exceptionally high affinity for other biologically active proteins, such as the mediators involved in inflammation. These therapeutic 'biological' molecules are genetically engineered to contain 'humanized' portions to limit the severe hypersensitivity reactions usually seen when mouse monoclonal antibodies were used. The first 'biologics' to reach clinical practice in IBD were anti-TNF-α monoclonal antibodies. TNF-α expression is strongly upregulated in inflamed segments of the gut mucosa in IBD and is also measurable systemically. Infliximab is a chimeric monoclonal antibody (i.e. the molecule is partly human and partly murine) that specifically binds and neutralizes endogenous TNF-α. Intravenous infusions of infliximab have been shown to be effective in both the induction and maintenance of remission in patients with CD and UC.

Problems with infliximab are often associated with its immunogenicity, and it has been shown that progressive lack of efficacy and some side-effects and infusion reactions are related to the presence of antibodies against the monoclonal antibody itself. Infusion reactions may occur after any number of infusions, and may be mitigated by the use of hydrocortisone and antihistamines at the time of the infusion, but may require cessation of the medication. In order to try to counter these problems other anti-TNF agents have been designed to try to have less immunogenicity. At present there is one additional anti-TNF drug licensed for use in IBD – adalimumab. This is a fully 'humanized' immunoglobulin, which means that whereas infliximab is about 75% human and 25% murine, adalimumab is 95% human. This has a theoretical benefit in terms of tolerability, as it may be less immunogenic. These differences are illustrated in Figure **11.2**. Certolizumab

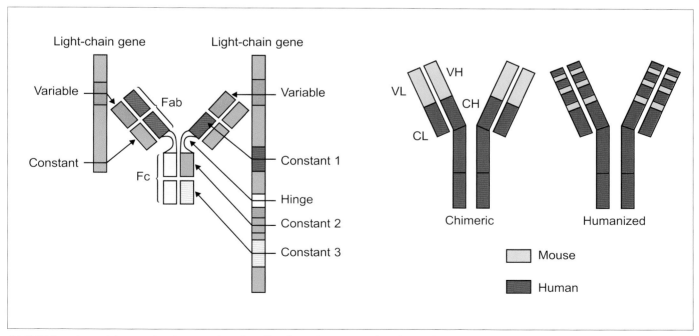

11.2 Chimeric and humanized monoclonal antibodies, demonstrating the reduced murine component in the humanized antibody.
VL: Variable region of the light chain; VH: variable region of the heavy chain; CL: constant region of the light chain; CH: constant region of the heavy chain.

pegol is a Fab′ fragment that comprises only the portion of antibody that interacts with antigen, and does not contain the Fc region. Certolizumab is also pegylated to promote prolonged and sustained release following subcutaneous administration. It has demonstrated some efficacy in clinical trials in CD, but there are not yet sufficient data for it to be licensed. Anti-TNF therapies are so effective at disabling this important mediator of the host immune system that there are concerns about whether patients treated with anti-TNF therapies are at excess risk of infection and malignancy. At present safety data are encouraging, but there are a number of issues that need to be borne in mind when prescribing these drugs.

There is clear evidence that anti-TNF therapy can lead to the reactivation of latent tuberculosis (TB). All patients in whom this therapy is contemplated should have a careful personal and family history taken, a chest radiograph to exclude evidence of TB, and if there is any concern a Mantoux or Heaf test before starting therapy.

Emerging reports suggest that serious infection is more likely in patients prescribed anti-TNF therapies concurrently with other immunosuppressive drugs including Aza, methotrexate, and corticosteroids. Anti-TNF treatment should be avoided in patients with active infection.

There have now been a small number of reports of a very rare form of lymphoma, hepatosplenic T cell lymphoma, in young Crohn's patients treated with infliximab. The age range is 12–32 years, and the disease is usually fatal. All these patients had also received Aza, and it is difficult to attribute the cause to a specific drug. However, in young patients concomitant biological and immunomodulator therapy should be used with caution and, if started, stopping Aza should probably be considered after 6 months. This short period may improve the efficacy of the infliximab by reducing immunogenicity, but there is evidence that prolonged therapy is not required. There are also important cost considerations when prescribing expensive biological therapies. The length of time that biological therapy should be continued is a matter for significant debate. Some authorities suggest it should be continued for the long term. Others, however, argue that in patients with no biological or clinical evidence of activity, the drugs should be stopped. Further research can be expected in this area.

Biological therapy is a rapidly changing and exciting development in the management of IBD. Emerging biological therapies that are being evaluated in IBD include adhesion molecule blocking antibodies, anti-T cell antibodies, and other anticytokine antibodies. Many of these are likely to reach the market in the next few years.

Chapter 12

Surgery in inflammatory bowel disease

Introduction

Despite the advances in medical therapy, surgery has an important role in both UC and CD. However, the indications for surgery and the operations performed differ substantially between the two conditions, and may also depend on the area of bowel affected.

Ulcerative colitis

Surgery may be considered in three major circumstances in UC:
- Acute severe UC.
- Chronic active UC with significant adverse effects on quality of life.
- Dysplastic lesions at colonoscopy or carcinoma.

Acute severe UC

Acute severe colitis is normally initially managed medically (see Chapter 5, Acute, severe colitis) with intravenous steroids, followed by ciclosporin or infliximab in non-responders. However, a proportion of patients will not respond to these second-line therapies and will require surgery. This can be a very substantial psychological shock for patients, particularly those who are newly diagnosed, and so it is important that they are introduced to a surgeon and stoma nurse early in the course of their hospital admission, so that they can become used to the possibility of surgery. The most important consideration in the timing of surgery for acute severe UC is not to persevere with medical therapies that are clearly ineffective, and the decision to operate should not generally be delayed for more than 1 week or 10 days after admission, as the chances of encountering complications of surgery increase dramatically as the patient becomes steadily less well, and has had increasing cumulative doses of corticosteroids. For patients who present with either overt perforation or toxic megacolon surgery should not be delayed, and should generally be undertaken immediately. In patients with toxic dilatation who are systemically otherwise well it is reasonable to try medical therapy for 24 hours, but if this is not effective they should proceed to colectomy. The typical appearance of a resected colon is shown in Figure **12.1**.

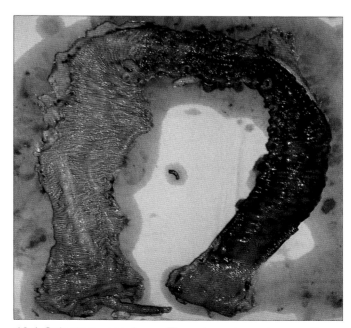

12.1 Colectomy specimen. There is a sharp demarcation in the mid-transverse with severe UC distal to this and essentially normal mucosa proximally.

Chronic active UC

Chronic active colitis is an indication for surgery if it is having a substantial impact on a patient's quality of life. This is particularly true for those patients who are either steroid dependent, and have accumulated significant side-effects, or those who are steroid resistant and do not respond to, or are intolerant of, second-line therapy such as Aza. For these patients surgery can reinstate a more normal quality of life, and can allow the patients to regain control of their symptoms.

Dysplastic lesions

The detection of malignancy, high-grade dysplasia at colonoscopic surveillance, or low-grade dysplasia in patients at high risk are indications for proctocolectomy in UC. There is currently debate over whether proctocolectomy is required in patients with polypoid dysplasia; in patients who have definitely normal mucosa adjacent to the polypoid area a more limited resection with close surveillance post-operatively may suffice. However, the risks of further dysplastic lesions should be discussed with the patient.

Operations for UC

Because of the likelihood of recurrence in the remaining bowel any surgery for UC involves colectomy. The mechanics of the surgery will depend on the indication, and the circumstances under which the surgery is performed. The final outcome can be either an end ileostomy or an ileal pouch–anal anastomosis, where the ileum is fashioned into a pouch which is anastomosed to the anus. This allows the patient to use the toilet in a normal fashion, but it should be noted that most patients with pouches use the toilet 5–8 times a day. This frequency is not associated with the debilitating urgency that characterizes UC. The major characteristics of bowel habit with a pouch are listed in *Table 12.1*.

Subtotal colectomy (*12.2*)

Subtotal colectomy is performed in the acute setting, when patients with acute severe UC have failed to respond to medical treatment or have colonic dilatation or perforation. In this operation the colon is excised, leaving a rectal stump *in situ*. The ileum is brought out onto the skin in the right iliac fossa as an ileostomy. This is the safest operation to perform in the unwell patient, and will allow the surgeon to fashion a pouch at a later stage, and finally to close the ileostomy a few months after that (three stage pouch procedure) – see 'panproctocolectomy and ileoanal pouch' below.

Panproctocolectomy and end-ileostomy

Patients who are undergoing elective or semielective procedures may opt to have the entire colon and rectum excised and an ileostomy formed. This is an irreversible operation, and has the advantages of curing the underlying UC and virtually eliminating the risk of developing colon cancer. However, this has to be weighed against the potential problems of managing a stoma.

Panproctocolectomy and ileoanal pouch

This can be done in either one, two, or three stages. As mentioned above the three stage procedure is undertaken for patients who require urgent subtotal colectomy for acute disease, and then subsequently undergo a modified two

Table 12.1 Characteristics of bowel habit in patients with ileoanal pouches

Function	Characteristics with a pouch
Average bowel motions/24 h	5–8
Average nocturnal bowel frequency	1/night
Patients with daytime faecal seepage	5%
Patients with nocturnal faecal seepage	8%
Patients using antidiarrhoeal medicines	35%

stage procedure. In the two stage procedure the rectum is excised and the ileoanal pouch formed and anastomosed, but in order to allow the anastomosis to heal a loop ileostomy is formed above it so that the anastomosis is not exposed to the faecal stream (**12.3**). At an interval of several months the ileostomy is then reversed, and the pouch allowed to function. In a one stage procedure the anastomosis is fashioned, and allowed to function immediately. This may work well in patients who are fit, and in whom the anastomosis is clearly sound; however, if there

12.2 Subtotal colectomy. The rectum is left *in situ*, whilst the remaining colon is resected and an ileostomy formed.

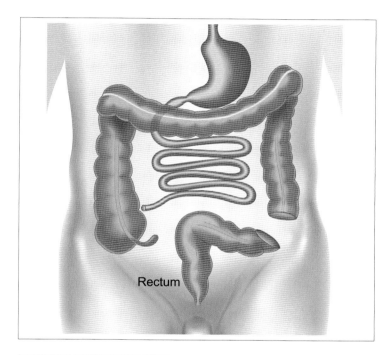

Rectum

12.3 Ileoanal pouch with covering ileostomy.

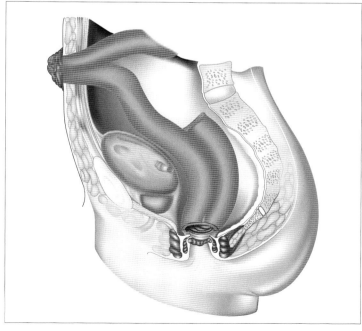

are problems with the anastomosis then the lack of a covering ileostomy can lead to more severe complications, and even to long-term pouch dysfunction. There are three major configurations of pouch design (**12.4**), the most commonly used of which is the J pouch (**12.5, 12.6**). It is normally stapled in place, which probably gives optimal functional results, although some surgeons prefer a hand sewn approach.

*Subtotal colectomy and ileorectal anastomosis (**12.7**)*
This operation is rarely performed in UC, but may be considered in the small minority of cases where the disease in the rectum is mild and/or quiescent. It has the disadvantage of leaving diseased colon behind, but if the disease is mild and controllable then the functional outcome from the rectum may be good, and possibly better than a pouch operation.

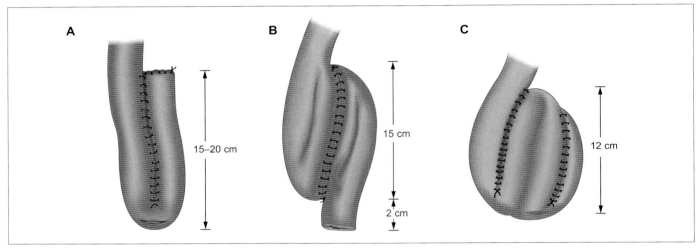

12.4 Configurations of ileoanal pouch. (**A**) J pouch; (**B**) S pouch; (**C**) W pouch.

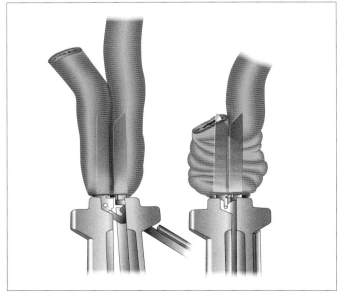

12.5 A stapled J pouch.

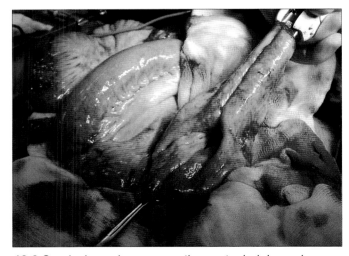

12.6 Surgical specimen – creating a stapled J pouch.

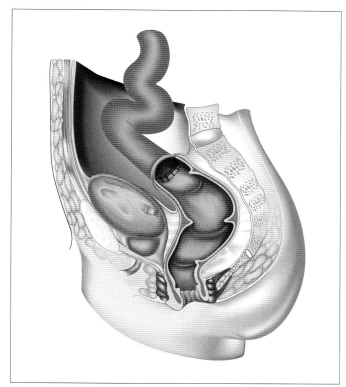

12.7 Subtotal colectomy and ileorectal anastomosis. The rectum is left in place and the ileum anastomosed to it. This is suitable only for the small minority of UC patients with relative rectal sparing.

Table 12.2 Complications of pouch surgery

Complication	Frequency (%)
Failure	7
Pouchitis	15–35
Fistula	9
Obstruction (small bowel)	9
Stricture	13

Complications of surgery for UC

Patients undergoing surgery for UC can develop all the complications associated with major surgery including adhesions leading to obstruction, infection in the wound, chest, or anastomosis, bleeding, and deep vein thrombosis. IBD patients may be more prone to all of these, particularly those with active disease, and if they have been on large doses of corticosteroids pre-operatively.

While most stomas work well problems may arise from stomas which either evert or invert, making adhesion of bags difficult. Incisional herniation at the site may also complicate stomas. If the outputs are persistently too high patients may become dehydrated, and may need to take supplemental electrolyte solutions such as St Mark's solution. In addition proton pump inhibitors may slow down secretions, and loperamide may slow gut transit and decrease stoma output.

The important specific complications of pouch surgery are summarized in *Table 12.2* and detailed below:

Pouch failure

In about 5–10% of patients the pouch simply does not function as well as it should. In some patients the pouch may need to be taken down, and may be refashioned, and in a small proportion (~2%) it may need to be excised completely and permanently.

Pouchitis

About 35% of patients will develop pouchitis (inflammation of the pouch). In most cases this is acute, and responds well to treatment with antibiotics, usually metronidazole or ciprofloxacin for 1 week. A minority of patients may develop more persistent inflammation – chronic pouchitis – and in these circumstances the treatment options are similar to those for the original UC – steroids, immune suppressants, and occasionally biological therapies. In these cases all patients should have an endoscopic examination of the pouch with histological confirmation, as stricturing at the anastomosis or in the pre-pouch ileum may produce similar symptoms.

Fistulae

These are rare, but pouch–vaginal fistulae can be difficult to treat, and if symptomatic may require surgical repair. In some cases the pouch may need to be completely revised. A pouch–vaginal fistula is illustrated in Figure **12.8**.

Fecundity

Female patients undergoing pouch surgery may have a significantly decreased chance of conceiving post-operatively. Estimates suggest that this decrease may be as much as 50%, and thus some patients may decide to have a family before undergoing restorative pouch surgery. In patients who become pregnant an elective Caesarean section should be considered in order to preserve the pouch function.

Surgery for CD

The role of surgery in CD is different from UC, partly because the disease nearly always recurs after surgery. This means that extensive resections should be avoided if at all possible in order to minimize the chances of running into problems due to a short gut. The major indications for surgery are:

Stricturing disease

Where there is a fibrous stricture causing obstructive symptoms medical therapy will not be successful, and surgery is required in order to alleviate the symptoms.

Fistulizing disease

Medical treatment of fistulizing disease is generally poor. Biological therapy and immune suppressants may have some effect, but even these often need to be used in combination with surgical therapy. The priority is to drain any pockets of infection, to lay open tracts, and to allow

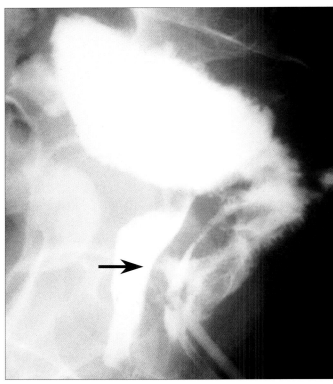

12.8 Pouch–vaginal fistula. The tract fills the vagina with dye introduced into the rectum (arrow).

healing while preserving free drainage (often by the insertion of Setons). In rare cases of severe perianal disease a proctectomy may be necessary to give the patient adequate quality of life.

Active disease

For active colonic disease which behaves like UC the surgical options are similar to those of UC, with the addition of the possibility of a defunctioning ileostomy as a means of resting the colon and allowing it to heal. In addition, for short segments of disease restricted to the ileocaecal region an ileocaecal resection may be an extremely effective therapy, and may be performed using a laparoscopically assisted approach.

Operations for CD

Strictureplasty (12.9)

This operation is effective for short fibrous strictures. It involves incising lengthways along the stricture and then closing the incision by suturing it horizontally. This

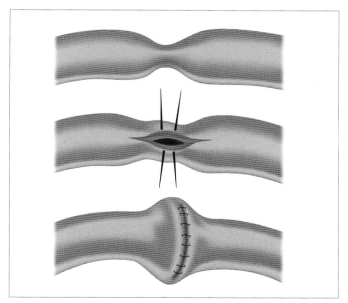

12.9 Strictureplasty. A short stricture is incised lengthways and sutured horizontally to increase the luminal diameter and alleviate symptoms.

increases the diameter of the lumen without removing any bowel. This has an advantage in terms of preservation of bowel length, but obviously means that the disease has not been resected, and thus adjunctive medical therapy may be required immediately post-operatively in order to maintain the symptomatic response. It may be a particularly useful technique in patients with multiple short strictures, where resection may mean the removal of large segments of bowel.

Limited resection

Classically limited resection is an ileocaecal resection of terminal ileal disease, but this may be performed on any isolated segment of CD. Ileocaecal resection is a very effective treatment for limited ileocaecal disease, and should be discussed with patients along with medical therapies. The question of medication to prevent post-operative recurrence is difficult. In patients who are undergoing a first operation there may be modest benefit to commencing 5-ASA therapy, and for a second or subsequent resection Aza therapy may be appropriate. There is also evidence for the use of metronidazole or ornidazole for 3 months post-operatively to reduce the risk of relapse. The latter is probably preferable due to the lower incidence of side-effects, particularly peripheral neuropathy.

Defunctioning or loop ileostomy

In patients with persistently active colonic CD defunctioning the colon by means of a loop ileostomy may induce some degree of healing. However, when the colon is rejoined the chances of relapse are high and 50% of patients will ultimately require a colectomy. A short period of defunctioning may also be useful in the treatment of patients with severe fistulizing disease in order to defunction the affected area of bowel, particularly with rectovaginal fistulae and other fistulae from gut to other organs.

Colectomy and proctocolectomy

The indications for these operations are similar to those in UC for patients who have severe colonic disease.

Drainage surgery

In fistulizing CD the key to management is the clearance of infection and the establishment of effective drainage. The best way of establishing what needs to be done is normally a combination of MRI of the pelvis and an examination under anaesthesia. This will allow the surgeon to explore all potential fistula tracts, to drain any collections, and perform fistulotomies on any simple fistulae. Noncutting Setons (knotted loops of large silk suture, silastic vessel markers, or rubber bands) may be placed in complex fistulae. These loops are designed to allow free drainage and to promote fibrosis. They may remain *in situ* for several months, until they either fall out or are removed. This approach can be used in combination with aggressive medical therapy once all the sepsis is drained, such as the use of biological therapy (infliximab or adalimumab). In severe cases where there is associated active rectal disease defunctioning the colon may aid in the healing of active disease (see above) and in extreme cases proctectomy may be required.

Repair surgery

Repair of fistulae is often unrewarding, particularly in the case of rectovaginal fistulae. In these cases surgical drainage succeeds in only 20% of cases. More aggressive surgery may be required with the use of advancement flaps to try and heal persistent large fistulae. However, even with this complex surgery success rates are low.

Complications of surgery for CD

As with surgery for UC (see above) CD patients are at risk of all the complications of major surgery, and often the presence of active inflammation and use of corticosteroids may increase these risks.

Wound dehiscence and fistula formation

In patients with fistulizing CD fistulae may form post-operatively, and in patients with active disease, particularly those on corticosteroid therapy, wound dehiscence may occur and may then lead to long-term fistula formation. Often these patients require the wound to be taken down and left to heal by secondary intention. This may necessitate a long in-patient stay.

Anastomotic leaks

These may occur in any form of surgery, but are particularly likely if diseased bowel has been used in an anastomosis either deliberately or unwittingly.

Short bowel syndrome

In patients who have had multiple resections and are left with less than 110–120 cm of bowel, problems may be encountered with absorbing sufficient nutrition to maintain a healthy nutritional status. These problems may manifest by the inability to maintain magnesium or calcium levels (with fitting or tetany) or other trace elements or by the failure to maintain body weight. Clearly the best approach is to try to avoid unnecessary bowel resections, but in some cases repeated resections are unavoidable. Supplemental nutrition may be given enterally using elemental or polymeric feeds or by overnight nasogastric feeding, but in some cases parenteral nutrition will be necessary. This requires careful training of all involved in order to ensure that the feeding lines are kept sterile, and the risk of line infection is minimized. For a small proportion of patients small bowel transplantation may be an appropriate option.

Recommended reading

Hanauer S and Bayless TM (eds). *Surgery for UC in Advanced Therapy of IBD*, BC Becker, Ontario, 2001.

Hanauer S and Bayless TM (eds). *Surgery for Crohn's disease in Advanced Therapy of IBD*, BC Becker, Ontario, 2001.

Index

MONKLANDS HOSPITAL
LIBRARY
MONKSCOURT AVENUE
AIRDRIE ML60JS
☎01236712005

MONACLONE LIBRARY
AIRDRIE NL6 0JS
☎ 01236712005